Keto Fat Bombs:

100+ Savory & Sweet Ketogenic Fat Bomb Recipes You Need To Try!

Kevin Moore © 2018

Disclaimer:

This book is for informational purposes only and the author, his agents, heirs, and assignees do not accept any responsibilities for any liabilities, actual or alleged, resulting from the use of this information.

This report is not "professional advice." The author encourages the reader to seek advice from a professional where any reasonably prudent person would do so. While every reasonable attempt has been made to verify the information contained in this eBook, the author and his affiliates cannot assume any responsibility for errors, inaccuracies or omissions, including omissions in transmission or reproduction.

Any references to people, events, organizations, or business entities are for educational and illustrative purposes only, and no intent to falsely characterize, recommend, disparage, or injure is intended or should be so construed. Any results stated or implied are consistent with general results, but this means results can and will vary. The author, his agents, and assigns, make no promises or guarantees, stated or implied. Individual results will vary and this work is supplied strictly on an "at your own risk" basis.

Introduction

Thanks for purchasing my book "Keto Fat Bombs: 100+ Savory & Sweet Ketogenic Fat Bomb Recipes You Need To Try!"

I hope you like all the recipes I've included. There are so many great fat bombs to try out on the keto diet. These quick and easy recipes should help get you started off on the right foot. Whether you like things savory or sweet this recipe guide has you covered.

Let's begin!

Chapter One: What Is A Keto Fat Bomb?

What Constitutes A Keto Fat Bomb?

1. Fat bombs are either sweet or savory. You'll find more recipes that swing towards the sweet side but there are plenty of savory recipe options available. A lot of the sweeter recipes call for stevia, a lower calorie and no-carb sweetener. Many of the savory fat bombs are made with items like bacon, chicken, sausage, or salmon.

2. Fat bombs are small in size. These items are high in fat so they are meant to be eaten in smaller-sized servings. They will normally take the shape of miniature muffins or a smaller-sized ball.

3. Fat bombs can be made in larger batches and stored in the refrigerator or freezer. Many fat bomb recipes make 10 or more servings at a time. Ideal for people who want to cook once or twice a week and still have healthy options on hand throughout the week. Fat bombs contain a high amount of fat and therefore will need to be kept cold when being stored. These items are not meant to sit at room temperature for long periods. Fat bombs can usually last for between 1 to 2 weeks when stored properly.

4. Fat bombs are high in healthy fats. These healthy fats are important when following a keto diet because they help to lower the levels of inflammation in the body. Many keto fat bombs will have some form of coconut butter or coconut oil in them. These oils also help to solidify the fat bombs and therefore make them less of a mess to eat.

5. Fat bombs will often have seeds or nuts. Nuts are only meant to be eaten in small amounts due to the number of carbohydrates they contain. This makes them ideal for fat bombs. Peanuts are not technically nuts so the keto diet substitutes peanut butter with almond butter in their recipes.

3 General Ingredients In Fat Bomb Recipes

1. Healthy Fats - These include coconut milk, coconut oil, coconut cream, bacon fat, butter, ghee, cacao butter, avocado oil.

2. Flavoring - These include cacao powder, peppermint, sugar-free vanilla extract, salt, dark chocolate, and spices.

3. Texture - These include pecans, cacao nibs, bacon bits, almonds, shredded coconut, chia seeds, and walnuts.

3 Steps For Making Fat Bombs

1. Mix each of your ingredients together in your mixing bowl, blender, or processor. Melt any solids that need to become liquid.

2. Form your fat bombs by hand or pour your mixture into a baking pan or muffin cups.

3. Freeze or refrigerate your fat bombs for a few hours until the mixture solidifies. Cut your fat bombs into slices if you made them in a baking pan.

Chapter Two: Sweet Keto Fat Bomb Recipes

In this section, I will show you 75+ sweet ketogenic fat bomb recipes you can cook for yourself. These are keto fat bombs are geared towards people wanting to satisfy their sweet tooth. These are easy to prepare no matter what your level in the kitchen. These tasty treats will help keep you on track with your ketogenic diet.

Almond Joy Fat Bombs (Serves 12)

Ingredients:

Coconut Filling:

1 cup of Unsweetened Coconut Flakes

2 tablespoons of Coconut Oil

1/4 cup of Unsweetened Coconut Milk

1/2 teaspoon of Almond Extract

1/4 teaspoon of Xanthan Gum

20 drops of Liquid Stevia

<u>*Chocolate Coating:*</u>

4 tablespoons of Coconut Oil

2 ounces of Unsweetened Bakers Chocolate

12 Almonds

20 drops of Liquid Stevia

<u>Directions:</u>

<u>*Coconut Filling:*</u>

1. Heat your saucepan over a low heat and add your coconut milk to your pan.

2. Add your coconut flakes and coconut oil, and stir allowing it to cook down a little.

3. Add the stevia drops and your almond extract. Stir and allow it to cook on low for approximately 5 minutes.

4. Add your xanthan gum and stir.

5. Line your 8x4 loaf pan with parchment paper and pour your coconut mixture into your pan. Press it out evenly over your parchment paper (1/2 inch thick) and allow it to set in the fridge for 1 hour.

6. Pull out your parchment paper and cut your coconut bar into 12 even-sized pieces.

7. Optional: Place your almond on top and press down gently into the center.

8. Place your almond joys in the freezer as you make your chocolate coating.

Chocolate Coating:

1. Chop your chocolate up and add to your microwave safe bowl.

2. Add your stevia and coconut oil to the bowl and microwave until fully melted.

3. Pull your almond joys out of the freezer and dip them into your chocolate coating either partially or fully coating them.

4. Keep stored in your refrigerator.

5. Serve and Enjoy!

Nutrition Facts:

Calories: 140.5

Calories from Fat: 128

Net Carbs: 1.5 grams

Almond Pistachio Fat Bombs (Serves 36)

Ingredients:

1 cup of Creamy Coconut Butter

1 cup of Coconut Oil (Firm)

1/2 cup of Finely Chopped & Melted Cacao Butter

1/4 cup of Chopped Raw Shelled Pistachios

1 cup of All-Natural Roasted Almond Butter

1/2 cup of Full Fat Coconut Milk (Chilled)

2 teaspoons of Chai Spice

1 tablespoon of Pure Vanilla Extract

1/4 cup of Ghee

1/4 teaspoon of Pure Almond Extract

1/4 teaspoon of Himalayan Salt

<u>Directions:</u>

1. Grease and line your 9-inch square baking pan with parchment paper. Leave some on a side for easier unmolding. Set to the side.

2. Melt your cacao butter in your small-sized saucepan set over a low heat, stirring often. Reserve.

3. Add all of your ingredients, except for shelled pistachios and cacao butter, to a large-sized mixing bowl. Mix with your hand mixer, starting on low speed and progressively moving higher until all of your ingredients are well combined and your mixture becomes airy and light.

4. Pour your melted cacao butter right into your almond mixture and mix on low speed until it's all incorporated.

5. Transfer to your prepared pan, spread as evenly as you can and sprinkle with your chopped pistachios.

6. Refrigerate until set, at least 4 hours but preferably overnight.

7. Cut into 36 even sized squares.

8. Serve and Enjoy!

<u>**Nutrition Facts:**</u>

Calories: 170

Calories from Fat: 157

Egg & Avocado Fat Bombs (Serves 5)

Ingredients:

1/2 Peeled Large Avocado (Seeds Removed)

3 Large Cooked Egg Yolks

1/4 cup of Mayonnaise

1/2 teaspoon of Salt

1 tablespoon of Lime or Lemon Juice

2 tablespoons of Chopped Spring Onions or Chives

Freshly Ground Black Pepper

Directions:

1. Cook your eggs.

2. Fill your small-sized saucepan with water up to three quarters. Add a pinch of salt. This will stop your eggs from cracking. Bring to a boil. Using your spoon or hand, dip each of your eggs in and out of the boiling water. This will stop your eggs from cracking as the temperature change won't be so sudden. To get your eggs hard-boiled it should take approximately 10 minutes. This timing works well for large-sized eggs. Once finished, remove from the heat and place in your bowl filled with cold water. When your eggs are chilled, peel off their shells.

3. Halve your avocado and remove the seeds and peel. Cut your eggs in half and carefully - without breaking your egg whites - spoon your egg yolks into a bowl.

4. Place your cut up avocado into your food processor and add your egg yolks, lemon juice, mayonnaise, pepper, and salt. Process until smooth. Alternatively, mash with your fork until creamy and well combined.

5. Serve with cucumber slices and spring onion on top, or fill up your egg white halves and make deviled eggs. To avoid browning, store in an airtight container and keep for a maximum of 5 days.

6. Enjoy!

Nutrition Facts:

Calories: 147

Net Carbs: 1.1 grams

Apple Pie Caramel Fat Bombs (Serves 24)

Ingredients:

2 Sliced & Cored Medium Organic Green Apples

2 tablespoons of Coconut Oil

1 teaspoon of Cinnamon

5.4 ounces of Coconut Cream

20 drops of English Toffee Stevia

1/2 cup of Coconut Butter

Pinch of Sea Salt

Directions:

1. In your skillet, saute your apples in the coconut oils until soft.

2. Add your cinnamon and stir to coat.

3. In your high-powered blender, combine the rest of your ingredients and blend on high until liquefied.

4. Pour into your silicone molds.

5. Place into your freezer until firm.

6. Pop out of your molds and store in a plastic bag in your refrigerator.

7. Serve and Enjoy!

Nutrition Facts:

Calories: 67

Carbs: 2.7 grams

Peanut Butter Chocolate Chip Cookie Dough Fat Bombs (Serves 12)

Ingredients:

6 ounces of Softened Cream Cheese

6 tablespoons of Softened Butter

3 tablespoons of Gentle Sweet (Equivalent of 1/4 cup of Sugar)

1 teaspoon of Vanilla Extract

6 scoops of Powdered MCT Oil

1/4 cup of Lily's Chocolate Chips

1/2 cup of Peanut Butter

Directions:

1. Combine your cream cheese, butter, cream cheese, vanilla extract, sweetener, and peanut butter in a bowl using your hand mixer. Mix them until well combined.

2. Stir in your chocolate chips. Cover and freeze for approximately 10 minutes.

3. Remove your bowl from your freezer and use a cookie scoop to scoop cookie dough onto a wax-paper lined dish.

4. Place your cookie dough balls back in the freezer for approximately 20 to 30 minutes, until firm.

5. Once frozen, remove your fat bombs from the freezer and place in a Ziploc bag or container. Store in your freezer until you're ready to eat.

6. Serve and Enjoy!

<u>Nutrition Facts:</u>

Calories: 214

Carbs: 6 grams

Coconut Chocolate Fat Bombs

<u>Ingredients:</u>

1/2 cup of Cocoa Powder

2 cups of Virgin Coconut Oil (Soft but Still Solid)

2 teaspoons of Vanilla Extract

6 tablespoons of Raw Honey

Dash of Salt (More to Taste)

<u>Directions:</u>

1. Add your cocoa powder, coconut oil, vanilla extract, honey, and salt to your food processor. Process until all of your ingredients are mixed evenly, stopping your food processor once or twice to scrape down the sides.

2. Taste your mixture to be sure that the flavor is to your liking. If desired, you can additional salt or honey as needed.

3. If using silicone molds, you want your coconut oil mixture to be pourable. If it's too thick, it's harder to fill your molds. You can process for longer to make your mixture thinner.

4. If you are not using molds, pick a flat surface that will fit in your freezer, such as a cutting board, and line it with your parchment paper. You want your mixture to be thicker and more solid, so it can be dropped onto your surface in individual dollops and won't run. If needed, you can put your food processor in the fridge for a couple of minutes to harden your mixture.

5. If using silicone molds, lay out your molds on your cutting board, then use your ladle to fill all of your molds with the coconut oil mixture.

6. If using a surface lined with parchment paper, use your spoon to drop dollops of your mixture onto your surface.

7. Transfer molds or surface to your freezer and freeze until your fat bombs become solid.

8. Pop them out and store in a lidded container in your freezer. Repeat this process until all of your fat bombs have been frozen.

9. These will keep in your freezer indefinitely. You can also store them in the refrigerator. Do not leave these at room temperature for more than a few minutes. Coconut oil melts at 76 degrees and these will get soft.

10. Serve and Enjoy!

Cinnamon Bun Fat Bombs (Serves 2)

Ingredients:

1/8 teaspoon of Cinnamon

1/2 cup of Unsweetened Creamed Coconut (Cut Into Chunks)

1st Icing:

1 tablespoon of Extra Virgin Coconut Oil (Not Melted)

1 tablespoon of Almond Butter

2nd Icing:

1/2 teaspoon of Cinnamon

1 tablespoon of Extra Virgin Coconut Oil or Almond Butter

Directions:

1. Line your dish or pan with appropriate liners.

2. In your bowl, using your hands, mix your cinnamon and coconut cream. Pat into the dish. Fills 2 mini loaf sections.

3. First Icing: In a different bowl using your whisk, whisk together your coconut oil and almond butter. Spread this over your creamed coconut. Place the bars in your freezer for approximately 5 to 8 minutes.

4. Second Icing: Using your whisk, mix your icing together in a bowl. Drizzle your icing over the bars.

5. Store in freezer until ready to serve.

6. Serve and Enjoy!

Chocolate Drizzled Coconut Oil Fat Bombs (Serves 14)

Ingredients:

2 cups of Shredded Unsweetened Coconut

4 ounces of Raw Dark Chocolate Chips

2 tablespoons of Raw Honey

1/3 cup of Melted Coconut Oil

1/2 tablespoon of Vanilla Bean Powder (Optional)

Directions:

1. In your blender, add your shredded coconut, raw honey, coconut oil, and vanilla bean powder. Blend until your mixture is fine and crumbled.

2. Line your small-sized baking sheet or plate with wax paper. Using your tablespoon-size measuring spoon, scoop mixture and form into small-sized mounds, using your hands. Set onto your wax paper.

3. Place in your freezer for approximately 10 minutes to set.

4. Using your double boiler, melt your chocolate until smooth.

5. Use a butter knife to drizzle your coconut bombs with chocolate. Place back into your refrigerator for approximately 10 minutes.

6. Store in your refrigerator until ready to serve.

7. Serve and Enjoy!

Coconut Berry Fat Bombs

Ingredients:

1/2 cup of Mixed Frozen Berries (Cherries, Raspberries, Strawberries, Blueberries, or Pomegranates)

1 cup of Virgin Coconut Oil

14 drops of Sweet Leaf Clear Liquid Stevia

1 teaspoon of Vanilla Extract

Directions:

1. Melt your coconut oil on your stove. While your oil is melting, briefly process your frozen fruit in a food processor so it's chopped up into small-sized pieces.

2. Add your stevia and vanilla extract to your food processor.

3. Pour your melted coconut oil into your food processor and process to mix with your fruit and other ingredients. Continue to mix until all of your fruit is smoothly blended into your oil.

4. The mixture should now be a thick blended consistency. If for some reason your mixture is still frozen and not blending properly, you can remove some of the frozen bits and melt them on your stove. Once melted, return your mixture to your food processor and try again to mix everything together smoothly.

5. Scoop the finished mixture into your molds or simply drop spoonfuls on your parchment paper-lined surface such as a cutting board.

6. Put your molds or parchment paper-lined surface into your freezer to firm up the fat bombs. After approximately 30 minutes, or whenever they become solid, remove from fat bombs from the molds or parchment paper and store in a container in your freezer.

7. Serve and Enjoy!

Craving Fighter Fat Bombs (Serves 32)

Ingredients:

1 cup of Melted Organic Coconut Oil

1 cup of Almond Butter (No Added Sugar)

1 cup of Organic Cacao Powder

Directions:

1. Melt your coconut oil and whisk in your cacao and almond butter until no lumps remain. Spoon 1/2 tablespoon of your mixture into each of your 32 small paper muffin cups.

2. Refrigerate or freeze until hard.

3. Store in your refrigerator.

4. Serve and Enjoy!

<u>Nutrition Facts:</u>

Calories: 123

Carbs: 2.25 grams

Fat: 11.75 grams

Sugar: 0.5 grams

Cheesecake Lemon Bombs (Serves 12)

Ingredients:

4 tablespoons of Softened Unsalted Butter

1/4 cup of Melted Coconut Oil

4 ounces of Softened Cream Cheese

1 teaspoon of Lemon Juice

1 tablespoons of Finely Grated Lemon Zest

Lemon Extract (Optional)

Stevia (To Taste)

Directions:

1. Blend all of your ingredients with your hand mixer until smooth.

2. Pour into your cupcake liners, tins, or molds.

3. Freeze until firm. At least a few hours but preferably overnight.

4. Sprinkle with your lemon zest.

5. Serve and Enjoy!

Nutrition Facts:

Calories: 105

Net Carbs: .25 grams

Pumpkin Pie Fat Bombs (Serves 24)

<u>Ingredients:</u>

1/2 cup of Coconut Oil

1 cup of Unsweetened Long Shredded Coconut

3/4 cup of Unsweetened Pumpkin Puree

1/4 teaspoon of Himalayan Rock Salt

1 1/2 teaspoons of Ground Ginger

1 tablespoon of Ground Cinnamon

1/4 teaspoon of Alcohol-Free Pure Vanilla Extract

25 drops of Alcohol-Free Stevia Extract

Pinch of Ground Cloves

1/4 cup of Grass-Fed Collagen (Optional)

Directions:

1. Line your baking sheet with two 12-count mini muffin silicone molds. Set to the side.

2. Add your shredded coconut, stevia, coconut oil, and salt to the bowl of your food processor. Process on high for approximately 5 to 8 minutes until drippy. You may have to remove your lid a couple of times and scrape the chunkier bits from the side of your bowl.

3. Once smooth, remove 1/4 cup of your coconut mixture, leaving your remaining coconut mix in your food processor bowl. Add your remaining ingredients and process until smooth again. If you use cold pumpkin puree, the coconut will harden. Just process until smooth again.

4. The texture of your pumpkin mixture will be similar to applesauce.

5. Divide your pumpkin mixture into your muffin cups. Press down until completely flat. Top with your reserved white coconut mixture. Transfer your baking sheet to the freezer and freeze for approximately 1 hour.

6. Serve and Enjoy!

Nutrition Facts:

Calories: 219

Calories From Fat: 182

Net Carbs: 2.4 grams

Sugars: 1.9 Grams

Chocolate Frozen Whips (Serves 12)

Ingredients:

4 tablespoons of Cocoa Powder

1 cup of Heavy Whipping Cream

1/2 teaspoon of Vanilla Extract

2 1/2 tablespoons of Swerve Sweetener

1 pinch of Sea Salt

Directions:

1. Put all your ingredients into your large-sized mixing bowl and beat on high with your whip attachment until the whipped cream has firm peaks.

2. Transfer your chocolate whipped cream to a piping bag fitted with a 1M piping tip.

3. On your parchment lined baking sheet swirl the whipped cream around into large mounds like soft serve ice cream. Make around 12 or so and freeze on your baking sheet for approximately 1 hour.

4. Store in a container and place in the freezer.

5. Serve and Enjoy!

<u>**Nutrition Facts:**</u>

Calories: 70

Net Carbs: 1.5 grams

Fudge Fat Bombs (Serves 30)

Ingredients:

1/2 cup of Unsweetened Cocoa Powder

1 cup of Almond Butter

1/3 cup of Coconut Flour

1 cup of Coconut Oil (Room Temperature)

1/4 teaspoon of Powdered Stevia

1/16 teaspoon of Pink Himalayan Salt

Directions:

1. Over a medium heat in your small-sized pot, melt and combine your almond butter and coconut oil.

2. In your same pot, add your dried ingredients and stir until well-combined.

3. Allow your mixture to cool slightly and taste test to determine if additional sweetener is needed.

4. Pour mixture into your bowl and place in freezer for approximately 90 minutes or pour into silicone mold (if you choose to use a silicone mold, skip steps #5 and #6 and just allow the fat bombs to solidify in freezer, approximately 3 to 4 hours).

5. Once solidified, remove the bowl from your freezer and form into balls.

6. Place your formed balls on a flat tray or plate and return to your freezer for approximately 15 to 20 minutes.

7. Serve and Enjoy!

Nutrition Facts:

Calories: 128

Net Carbs: 1.4 grams

Ginger Fat Bombs (Serves 10)

Ingredients:

3 ounces of Softened Coconut Oil

3 ounces of Softened Coconut Butter

1 teaspoon of Granulated Sweetener

1/4 cup of Unsweetened Shredded Coconut

1 teaspoon of Ginger Powder

Directions:

1. Mix all your ingredients in a pouring jug until your sweetener is dissolved.

2. Pour mixture into your silicone molds or ice block trays and refrigerate for approximately 10 to 15 minutes.

3. Serve and Enjoy!

<u>Nutrition Facts:</u>

Calories: 120

Carbs: 2.2 grams

Fat: 12.8 grams

Cashew & Cacao Fat Bombs (Serves 20)

Ingredients:

1 cup of Almond Butter

1 cup of Coconut Oil

1/2 cup of Cacao Powder

1/4 cup of Coconut Flour

1 cup of Raw Cashews

Directions:

1. In your non-stick medium saucepan over a medium heat, heat your coconut oil, and almond butter until mixed evenly, stirring often.

2. Pour your oil mixture from the pan into your bowl and mix in coconut flour and cacao powder.

3. Place your bowl in your freezer for approximately 15 minutes until your mixture cools and is solid.

4. While your mixture is cooling, place your cashews in a food processor and pulse lightly for a chopped texture.

5. When your coconut mixture is solidified, take 1/2 tablespoon of your mixture from the bowl, roll into a ball, and dip in the blended cashews.

6. Place your fat bombs on a plate. Repeat until you have used all of your mixture.

7. Refrigerate the fat bombs for approximately 5 minutes.

8. Make sure to store your leftover fat bombs in the refrigerator, otherwise they will melt quickly.

9. Serve and Enjoy!

Nutrition Facts:

Calories: 217

Carbs: 6.6 grams

Fat: 20.7 grams

Pecan Pie Clusters

Ingredients:

1 cup of Chopped Pecans

3 tablespoons of Butter

2 ounces of Chopped Dark or Sugar Free Chocolate

2 tablespoons of Zen Sweet

1/4 cup of Heavy Cream

1 teaspoon of Vanilla

Directions:

1. Over a medium heat, brown your butter until golden. Stir frequently being careful not to burn.

2. Once golden, add your heavy cream and whisk together. Turn down heat to a simmer.

3. Whisking quickly, add your sweetener and vanilla, being sure to break up any lumps.

4. Continue whisking occasionally for approximately 5 minutes as your mixture begins to thicken.

5. Mixture will have consistency similar to caramel and slightly darken. Remove from the heat.

6. Mix in your chopped pecans and spoon clusters onto parchment lined tray or plate.

7. Place in freezer for approximately 5 minutes.

8. Microwave your dark chocolate for 20 to 40 seconds until melted and smooth. Drizzle over clusters.

9. Serve and Enjoy!

<u>Nutrition Facts:</u>

Calories: 140

Carbs: 1 gram

Peppermint Coffee Fat Bombs (Serves 12)

Ingredients:

4 tablespoons of Coconut Oil

1/4 cup of Ghee

6 squares of 100% Cacao Unsweetened Chocolate Premium Baking Bar

2 teaspoons of Peppermint Extract

36 to 48 drops of Liquid Stevia (to taste)

2 tablespoons of Heavy Whipping Cream

Directions:

1. Melt your ghee and coconut oil in your microwave safe bowl.

2. Add in six squares of 100% Cacao Unsweetened Chocolate Premium Baking Bar Chocolate and heat for 30 second intervals until melted.

3. After your oil and chocolate is melted add your peppermint extract and liquid stevia and pour your mixture into mini silicone baking cups.

4. Place chocolate cups into your freezer for at least one hour or more until frozen.

5. Optional: Place one fat bomb into a coffee cup and brew coffee over your fat bomb. Froth 2 tablespoons of heavy whipping cream and add to your coffee.

6. Serve and Enjoy!

Nutrition Facts:

Calories: 115

Net Carbs: 2 grams

Key Lime Pie Fat Bombs (Serves 30)

Ingredients:

3/4 cup of Key Lime Juice

2 cups of Raw Cashews (Boiled for 12 minutes or Soaked for 2 hours)

1/2 cup of Coconut Butter

1 cup of Melted Coconut Oil

1/4 teaspoon of Powdered Stevia

Directions:

1. Combine all of your ingredients in your food processor and blend until well combined.

2. Transfer your mixture to a medium-sized bowl and place in freezer for approximately 20 to 30 minutes to cool.

3. Remove the mixture from your freezer and form into balls.

4. Place the balls in your freezer for approximately 20 minutes to harden. Place on a cookie sheet or plate lined with parchment paper to avoid the bottoms sticking.

5. Remove from your freezer once solid. Store in an airtight container in the refrigerator or freezer.

6. Serve and Enjoy!

<u>Nutrition Facts:</u>

Calories: 153

Carbs: 4 grams

Maple Almond Fudge Fat Bombs (Serves 24)

Ingredients:

1/2 cup of All Natural Almond Butter

1/4 cup of Butter

2 tablespoons of Coconut Oil

1 tablespoon of Sugar-Free Zero-Carb Maple Syrup

Directions:

1. Melt your almond butter, butter, and coconut oil in the microwave for approximately 2 minutes, stirring every 30 seconds, or until smooth and fully melted together.

2. Whisk in your maple syrup and stir well to combine.

3. Pour your mixture into bite-sized paper liners set inside a mini muffin tin.

4. Refrigerate or freeze until hardened.

5. You may store these at room temperature for a soft consistency or in the freezer or fridge for a firmer consistency.

6. Serve and Enjoy!

<u>Nutrition Facts:</u>

Calories: 58

Carbs: 1.5 grams

Mocha Ice Bombs (Serves 12)

Ingredients:

Mocha Ice Bombs:

1 cup of Cream Cheese or Mascarpone

2 tablespoons of Cocoa Unsweetened

4 tablespoons of Powdered Sweetener

4 tablespoons of Strong Coffee (Chilled)

Chocolate Coating:

2/3 cup of Melted 90% Chocolate

1/3 cup of Melted Cocoa Butter

Directions:

1. Mocha ice bombs can be made in your food processor, or in your mixing bowl using a hand blender.

2. Add your coffee to your cream cheese, cocoa, and sweetener.

3. Pulse or blend until smooth.

4. Roll about 2 tablespoons of your mocha ice bomb mixture and place them onto a tray or plate lined with baking parchment.

5. Mix your melted chocolate and cocoa butter together.

6. Roll each mocha ice bomb in your chocolate coating and place back on your lined plate.

7. Place in your freezer for approximately 2 hours, or until set.

8. Serve and Enjoy!

Nutrition Facts:

Calories: 127

Carbs: 2.2 grams

Raspberry Almond Chocolate Fat Bombs (Serves 8)

Ingredients:

1/2 cup of Coconut Butter

1/4 cup of Almond Butter

1/4 cup of Raw Almonds

1 tablespoon of Unsweetened Cocoa Powder

1/4 cup of Walnuts

1/4 teaspoon of Stevia Powder

1/4 cup of Frozen Raspberries

Directions:

1. In your bowl, mix together your coconut butter, stevia powder, almond butter, and cocoa powder.

2. Chop your walnuts and almonds.

3. Microwave your raspberries for approximately 40 to 60 seconds.

4. Place your parchment paper over a square pan and pour your chocolate butter inside. Sprinkle the nuts over and cover with your melted raspberries.

5. Place in the freezer for approximately one hour to freeze. Take it out and break it into 8 pieces.

6. Always keep frozen. You can transfer the chocolate pieces to a container after it's frozen.

7. Serve and Enjoy!

Nutrition Facts:

Calories: 82

Carbs: 3.1 grams

Samoa Fudge Fat Bombs (Serves 10)

Ingredients:

2 1/2 tablespoons of Melted Butter

3 1/2 tablespoons of Unsweetened Cocoa Powder

3 1/2 tablespoons of Swerve Sweetener

2 1/2 tablespoons of Melted Coconut Oil

2 tablespoons of Heavy Cream or Unsweetened Coconut Milk

Caramel Coating Ingredients:

2 1/2 tablespoons of Butter

2 tablespoons of Heavy Cream

2 1/2 tablespoons of Erythritol Swerve Sweetener

1/8 teaspoon of Vanilla Extract

1/8 teaspoon of Molasses or Low-Carb Maple Syrup

1 tablespoons of Unsweetened Fine Shredded Coconut

Directions:

1. In your large-sized mixing bowl combine all your fudge bomb ingredients. Mix together thoroughly. Pour or spoon your mixture into a lightly greased candy mold, ice cube tray, or cake pop pan.

2. Freeze for approximately 15 minutes or until firm.

3. In a small-sized saucepan over a medium heat melt your 2 1/2 tablespoons of butter for your caramel coating.

4. Once melted add your 2 1/2 tablespoons of sweetener, 2 tablespoons of heavy cream, and 1/8 teaspoon of molasses. Stir and heat until bubbling. Remove from the heat and stir in 1/8 teaspoon of vanilla extract. Let your caramel sauce rest for a couple minutes until it thickens.

5. Remove your fudge bombs from the freezer and place on your baking sheet lined with parchment paper or wax paper.

6. Drizzle or spoon your caramel sauce over truffle bombs and sprinkle with your shredded coconut.

7. Store in a covered container in the refrigerator or freezer.

8. Serve and Enjoy!

<u>**Nutrition Facts:**</u>

Calories: 102

Net Carbs: 1 gram

Sea Salt Chocolate Fat Bombs (Serves 10)

Ingredients:

1/2 cup of Heavy Whipping Cream

1/2 cup of Sunflower Butter

1 teaspoon of Vanilla

2 tablespoons of Cocoa Powder

1/2 cup of Coconut Oil

1 teaspoon of Cinnamon

1/3 cup of Cream Cheese

2 teaspoons of Coarse Sea Salt

3 tablespoons of Grass-Fed Butter

Directions:

1. Whip your heavy whipping cream until soft peaks form. Add your vanilla and fold in.

2. Place sunflower butter, grass-fed butter, cream cheese, coconut oil, cinnamon, and cocoa powder into the bowl of your food processor and process until smooth.

3. Gently fold your sunflower butter mixture into whipped cream until well combined.

4. Pipe mixture into silicone molds then sprinkle with coarse sea salt and freeze approximately 6 to 8 hours or overnight.

5. Serve and Enjoy!

Blueberry Cream Fat Bombs (Serves 30)

Ingredients:

4 ounces of Soft Goat Cheese

1/2 cup of Pecans

1/2 cup of Fresh Blueberries

1/2 teaspoons of Stevia

1 teaspoon of Vanilla Extract

1 cup of Almond Flour

1/4 cup of Unsweetened Shredded Coconut

Directions:

1. Process all your ingredients in a food processor until well combined.

2. Roll mixture into 30 small fat bombs.

3. Pour your coconut flakes into a small-sized bowl and lightly roll each fat bomb in your shredded coconut.

4. Serve and Enjoy!

<u>**Nutrition Facts:**</u>

Calories: 48

Net Carbs: 1 gram

Coconut Cinnamon Fat Bombs (Serves 10)

<u>Ingredients:</u>

1 cup of Coconut Milk (Full Fat & Canned)

1/2 teaspoon of Nutmeg

1 teaspoon of Vanilla Extract

1 teaspoon of Stevia Powder Extract

1/2 teaspoon of Cinnamon

1 cup of Coconut Butter

1 cup of Coconut Shreds

<u>Directions:</u>

1. Place a glass bowl over a saucepan with a few inches of water in it to create a double boiler.

2. Place all your ingredients except shredded coconut in a double boiler over a medium heat.

3. Mix your ingredients while waiting for them to melt.

4. When all your ingredients are combined remove the bowl from your heat.

5. Place your bowl in the fridge until it is hard enough to roll into balls, approximately 30 minutes.

6. Roll your contents into 1-inch balls and roll them through your coconut shreds.

7. Place your balls on a plate and refrigerate for one hour.

8. Keep refrigerated when not serving.

9. Serve and Enjoy!

<u>Nutrition Facts:</u>

Calories: 341

Net Carbs: 5.4 grams

Sweet Treat Chocolate Fat Bombs (Serves 4)

Ingredients:

2 ounces of Coconut Oil

1 teaspoon of Cocoa Powder

1 ounces of Cream Cheese

2 ounces of Dark Chocolate

1/2 ounces of Torani Sugar Free Vanilla Syrup

2 ounces of Almond Butter

8 drops of EZ-Sweetz

Directions:

1. Combine all of your items except the almond butter and microwave for approximately 30 seconds.

2. Stir your ingredients, if your chocolate is not fully melted, microwave again and continue to stir.

3. Pour a base layer into the mold that you're using.

4. Use a spoon and place a dollop of almond butter in the center.

5. Fill the rest of the mold to the top.

6. Freeze until the chocolate hardens. Once hard push them out of the mold.

7. Store in the refrigerator.

8. Serve and Enjoy!

Nutrition Facts:

Calories: 298

Net Carbs: 4 grams

Pudding Fat Bombs (Serves 6)

Ingredients:

1 box of Sugar-Free Jell-O Instant Pudding (Any Flavor)

3 cups of Heavy Whipping Cream

Directions:

1. Follow the instructions listed on the instant pudding box substituting the whipping cream for milk.

2. Store in the refrigerator once finished.

3. Serve and Enjoy!

Nutrition Facts:

Calories: 197

Net Carbs: 11 grams

Strawberry Shortcake Keto Fat Bombs (Serves 25)

<u>Ingredients:</u>

3/4 cup of Almond Flour

1/4 cup of Shredded Coconut

1/4 cup of Coconut Flour

1 teaspoon of Vanilla Extract

1/2 cup of Strawberries

1 teaspoon of Stevia

1 tablespoon of Coconut Oil

<u>Directions:</u>

1. Add all of your ingredients to a food processor and process until well combined.

2. Roll into 25 individual bites. If desired, roll in your shredded coconut.

3. Chill in the refrigerator for at least 1 hour.

4. Serve and Enjoy!

<u>Nutrition Facts:</u>

Calories: 34

Carbs: 2 grams

Fat: 2 grams

Coconut Orange Creamsicle Fat Bombs (Serves 10)

<u>Ingredients:</u>

1/2 cup of Coconut Oil

4 ounces of Cream Cheese

1/2 cup of Heavy Whipping Cream

10 drops of Liquid Stevia

1 teaspoon of Orange Vanilla Mio

<u>Directions:</u>

1. Measure out your coconut oil, heavy cream, and cream cheese.

2. Use an immersion blender to blend together all of your ingredients. If you're having a hard time blending the ingredients, you can microwave them for 30 seconds to 1 minute to soften them up.

3. Add your orange vanilla mio and liquid stevia into the mixture. Mix together with a spoon.

4. Spread your mixture into a silicone tray and freeze for approximately 2 to 3 hours.

5. Once hardened, remove from your silicone tray and store in your freezer.

6. Serve and Enjoy!

Nutrition Facts:

Calories: 178

Net Carbs: 1 gram

Chocolate Peanut Butter Fat Bombs (Serves 8)

Ingredients:

2 tablespoons of Heavy Cream

1/2 cup of Coconut Oil

6 tablespoons of Shelled Hemp Seeds

1/4 cup of Cocoa Powder

4 tablespoons of PB Fit Powder

1/4 cup of Unsweetened Shredded Coconut

1 teaspoon of Vanilla Extract

28 drops of Liquid Stevia

Directions:

1. Mix together all of your dry ingredients with the coconut oil. It will eventually turn into a paste.

2. Add vanilla, heavy cream, and liquid stevia. Mix again until everything is combined and slightly creamy.

3. Measure out unsweetened shredded coconut on to your plate.

4. Roll balls out using your hand and then roll in the unsweetened shredded coconut. Lay on to a baking tray covered with parchment paper. Set in the freezer for approximately 20 minutes.

5. Serve and Enjoy!

Nutrition Facts:

Calories: 210

Net Carbs: 1 gram

Cookie Dough Keto Fat Bombs (Serves 30)

Ingredients:

2 cups of Almond Flour

8 tablespoons of Softened Butter

1/2 teaspoon of Pure Vanilla Extract

1/3 cup of Swerve

2/3 cup of Lily's Dark Chocolate Chips

1/2 teaspoon of Kosher Salt

Directions:

1. In a large-sized bowl using a hand mixer, beat butter until light and fluffy. Add your vanilla, sugar, and salt and beat until well combined.

2. Slowly beat in your almond flour until no dry spots remain, then fold in your chocolate chips. Cover bowl with plastic wrap and place in your refrigerator to firm slightly approximately 15 to 20 minutes.

3. Using a small cookie scoop, scoop dough into small-sized balls. Store in your refrigerator if planning to eat within the week, or in the freezer for up to 1 month.

4. Serve and Enjoy!

Chocolate Walnut Fat Bombs (Serves 30)

Ingredients:

3 1/2 ounces of Dark Chocolate (85% Cocoa Solids)

1/3 cup of Small Walnut Pieces

1/4 cup of Coconut Oil

8 drops of Stevia

1 teaspoon of Cinnamon

Directions:

1. Melt your chocolate and coconut oil.

2. Crush your walnuts until you have small pieces.

3. Add your stevia, crushed walnuts, and cinnamon to your melted chocolate and coconut oil mix.

4. Pour into silicone molds or ice cube tray and freeze for approximately 5 minutes until the tops are set.

5. Remove from your freezer and press the larger walnut pieces on top.

6. Place in the refrigerator for approximately 20 minutes until your fat bombs have set.

7. Serve and Enjoy!

<u>Nutrition Facts:</u>

Calories: 46

Carbs: 0.7 grams

Fat: 4.8 grams

Everything Bagel and Lox Fat Bombs (Serves 36)

Ingredients:

4 ounces of Wild Caught Smoked Salmon

8 ounces of Organic Cultured Cream Cheese

2 Thinly Sliced Medium Scallions

Homemade Everything Bagel Seasoning

Directions:

1. Using a hand or stand mixer, beat cream cheese until fluffy.

2. Add your chopped smoked salmon and thinly sliced scallions.

3. Beat until well incorporated.

4. Roll into bite-sized balls then lightly coat in Everything Bagel Seasoning.

5. Chill 2 to 3 hours.

6. Serve and Enjoy!

<u>Nutrition Facts:</u>

Calories: 25

Carbs: 0.5 grams

Fat: 2 grams

Ice Cream Fat Bombs (Serves 5)

Ingredients:

4 Whole Pastured Eggs

4 Yolks From Pastured Eggs

2 teaspoons of Vanilla Bean Powder

1/3 cup of Melted Cacao Butter

1/3 cup of Xylitol or 15 to 20 drops of Alcohol-Free Stevia

1/3 cup of Melted Coconut Oil

1/4 cup of MCT Oil

8 to 10 Ice Cubes

Directions:

1. Add all ingredients but ice cubes into your high powered blender. Blend on high for approximately 2 minutes, until creamy.

2. While your blender is still running, remove the top portion of the lid and drop in 1 ice cube at a time, allowing your blender to run about 10 seconds between each ice cube. The goal here is to dilute the mixture just a bit and make it cold so it will run through the ice cream maker easier.

3. Once all of your ice has been added, pour your cold mixture into your ice cream maker and churn on high for approximately 20 to 30 minutes, depending on your ice cream maker. If you do not have an ice cream maker, transfer the mixture to your 9x5 loaf pan and place in your freezer. Set the timer for 30 minutes before taking out to stir. Repeat for 2 to 3 hours, until desired consistency is met.

4. Serve immediately as soft-serve or scoop into a 9x5 loaf pan and freeze for approximately 45 minutes. Store covered in the freezer for up to 1 week.

5. Enjoy!

<u>Nutrition Facts:</u>

Calories: 430

Net Carbs: 1.8 grams

Chocolate Chip Cookie Dough Fat Bombs (Serves 24)

Ingredients:

1 stick of Softened Unsalted Butter

8 ounces of Softened Cream Cheese

1/2 cup of Golden Monk Fruit Sweetener

1/2 cup of Crunchy Almond Butter

2 ounces of 100% Cacao Baker's Chocolate Bar

Directions:

1. In your mixing bowl, using an electric mixer, mix all of your ingredients excluding chocolate until well-combined.

2. Refrigerate your mixture for 30 minutes.

3. In your food processor, pulse your chocolate until broken into small-sized pieces.

4. Remove your mixing bowl from the refrigerator. Fold in your chocolate pieces, and form your mixture into balls or scoop and flatten into a silicone mold. (If forming fat bombs into balls, line your plate with parchment paper and set fat bombs on top of the parchment paper.)

5. Harden the fat bombs in your freezer for approximately 45 minutes.

6. Serve and Enjoy!

<u>Nutrition Facts:</u>

Calories: 98

Net Carbs: 1.2 grams

Pumpkin Spice Fat Bombs (Serves 24)

Ingredients:

4 ounces of Softened Cream Cheese

1/2 cup of Pecans

2 teaspoons of Pumpkin Pie Spice

1/2 cup of Pumpkin Puree

1/2 cup of Coconut Oil

1/4 cup of Golden Monk Fruit Sweetener

1/4 teaspoon of Cinnamon

Avocado Oil Cooking Spray

Directions:

1. In your small-sized pan over a medium heat, spray your avocado oil cooking spray and toast the pecans until fragrant. Remove from heat and set to the side to cool.

2. In your medium-sized pot over a medium-low heat, melt your coconut oil and cream cheese until well combined.

3. Pour your coconut oil and cream cheese mixture into a medium-sized bowl and add your pumpkin puree, pumpkin pie spice, and monk fruit sweetener. Mix together using your electric hand mixer.

4. Scoop your mixture into a silicone mold, top with your toasted pecans, and sprinkle with cinnamon.

5. Place your silicone mold in a freezer and freeze until solid, approximately 4 hours.

6. Pop your fat bombs out of the silicone mold.

7. Serve and Enjoy!

<u>Nutrition Facts:</u>

Calories: 78

Net Carbs: 1 gram

Pecan Pie Fat Bombs (Serves 18)

Ingredients:

1 1/2 cups of Pecans

1/4 cup of Coconut Butter

1/2 cup of Shredded Coconut

2 tablespoons of Flax Meal

2 tablespoons of Chia Seeds

2 tablespoons of Hemp Seeds

2 tablespoons of Pecan Butter

1 teaspoon of Vanilla Bean Ghee

1/2 teaspoon of Vanilla Bean Powder or Vanilla Extract

1 1/2 teaspoons of Cinnamon

1/4 teaspoon of Kosher Salt

Directions:

1. In the bowl of your food processor, combine all of your ingredients. Pulse for approximately 1 to 2 minutes, until the mixture starts to break down. It will first become powdery and will stick together, but still be crumbly.

2. Keep processing until the oils start to release a bit and the mixture sticks together easily. Be careful not to over process or you'll have nut butter.

3. Use a small-sized cookie scoop or a tablespoon scoop to divide your mixture into equal pieces. Use your hands to roll into balls and place on a plate or baking sheet and place in your refrigerator to firm up for approximately 30 minutes.

4. Store in an airtight container in your refrigerator or freezer.

5. Serve and Enjoy!

Nutrition Facts:

Calories: 120

Carbs: 3.8 grams

White Chocolate Raspberry Fat Bombs (Serves 12)

<u>Ingredients:</u>

1/2 cup of Freeze-Dried Raspberries

1/2 cup of Coconut Oil

1/4 cup of Swerve

2 ounces of Cacao Butter

<u>Directions:</u>

1. Line your 12-cup muffin pan with paper liners or use a silicone muffin pan.

2. Heat your coconut oil and cacao butter in your small-sized saucepan over a low heat until melted. Remove your pan from the heat.

3. Grind the freeze-dried raspberries in your food processor or blender.

4. Add your pulverized berries and sweetener to your saucepan. Stir until your sweetener is mostly dissolved.

5. Divide your mixture among the muffin cups. The raspberry powder will sink to the bottom. Stir your mixture as you pour it into each mold so each muffin cup has raspberry powder.

6. Chill for 1 hour or until firm. They'll keep in the refrigerator for a few weeks.

7. Serve and Enjoy!

Nutrition Facts:

Calories: 153

Net Carbs: 1.2 grams

Chocolate Coconut Almond Fat Bombs (Serves 30)

Ingredients:

1/2 cup of Melted Coconut Oil

1/4 cup of Cacao Powder or Cocoa Powder

1/2 cup of Melted Coconut Butter

1/2 teaspoon of Vanilla Extract

1 teaspoon of Almond Extract

1/4 cup of Crushed Sliced Almonds

1/4 cup of Unsweetened Finely Shredded Coconut

10 drops of Stevia (or 1/2 teaspoon of Erythritol)

1/4 cup of Cacao Nibs

Directions:

1. Mix your almond extract, coconut oil, cacao powder, coconut butter, stevia, and vanilla extract together. If using erythritol: heat in the microwave or on a stove for 1 to 2 minutes until the erythritol is dissolved.

2. Add your crushed slivered almonds, cacao nibs, and coconut flakes. With a tablespoon, fill your mini cupcake liners or an ice cube tray, putting 1 tablespoonful in each. Store in your refrigerator.

3. Serve and Enjoy!

Nutrition Facts:

Calories: 72

Carbs: 1 gram

Fat: 7 grams

Layered Peppermint Patties Fat Bombs (Serves 24)

Ingredients:

1/2 cup of Coconut Butter

2 tablespoons of Coconut Oil

1/4 cup of Unsweetened Shredded Coconut

4 ounces of 100% Dark Chocolate

1 teaspoon of Peppermint Extract

4 tablespoons of Coconut Oil

Stevia

Directions:

1. Soften your coconut butter and 2 tablespoons of coconut oil and mix together with your unsweetened shredded coconut, stevia, and peppermint extract.

2. Spoon 2 teaspoons into each of your mini muffin cups and set in the refrigerator for approximately 1 hour. Check this layer is solid before proceeding to the next step.

3. Melt 4 tablespoons of coconut oil and dark chocolate and mix together well. Spoon 1 teaspoon into each mini muffin cup so that it forms a layer. Set in your refrigerator for approximately 1 hour. Check this layer is solid before going to the next step.

4. You can repeat steps 2 and 3 for as many layers as you want.

5. Serve and Enjoy!

Nutrition Facts:

Calories: 100

Net Carbs: 2 grams

Vanilla Fat Bombs Dipped In Chocolate Fat Bombs (Serves 16)

<u>Ingredients:</u>

1/4 cup of 100% Dark Chocolate

1 cup of Coconut Butter

1 cup of Unsweetened Shredded Coconut

1 cup of Coconut Milk

1 tablespoon of Vanilla Extract

Stevia

<u>Directions:</u>

1. Melt your coconut butter and the coconut milk in a saucepan over a low heat.

2. Add in all of your ingredients except for the dark chocolate into your saucepan.

3. Mix together well. Let your mixture cool in the refrigerator for approximately 1 to 2 hours.

4. Then form small balls from your mixture (approximately 15 to 20). Place your balls into the refrigerator to solidify for 2 to 3 hours.

5. Melt your dark chocolate (in the microwave or on the stove).

6. Dip each of your balls into the chocolate, and place your dipped balls onto the parchment paper. Place back into your refrigerator.

7. Serve and Enjoy!

<u>Nutrition Facts:</u>

Calories: 180

Net Carbs: 3 grams

Chocolate Almond Fat Bombs (Serves 15)

Ingredients:

1 cup of Coconut Oil

1 cup of Almond Butter

1/4 cup of Coconut Flour

1/2 cup of Cacao Powder

10 to 15 Whole Almonds

Stevia

Directions:

1. Melt your almond butter and coconut oil in a saucepan. Add in your cacao powder, stevia, and coconut flour and mix together well.

2. Let your mixture cool and then form 10 to 15 small-sized balls from your mixture.

3. Stick an almond into the middle of each.

4. Refrigerate to set and store in your refrigerator.

5. Serve and Enjoy!

Nutrition Facts:

Calories: 260

Net Carbs: 3 grams

Fudge Macadamia Chocolate Fat Bombs (Serves 6)

Ingredients:

4 ounces of Chopped Macadamias

2 ounces of Cocoa Butter

2 tablespoons of Swerve

2 tablespoons of Unsweetened Cocoa Powder

1/4 cup of Heavy Cream or Coconut Oil

Directions:

1. Melt your cocoa butter in your small-sized saucepan in a bath of water. (I just use another slightly bigger saucepan, half full of water)

2. Add cocoa powder to your saucepan.

3. Add the swerve and mix well until all your ingredients are well blended and melted.

4. Add the macadamias and stir in well.

5. Add your cream, mix well and bring back to temperature.

6. Now pour in your molds or paper candy cups.

7. Allow it to cool, then put in the refrigerator to harden.

8. Keep at room temperature, with a slightly softer consistency than chocolate.

9. Serve and Enjoy!

<u>Nutrition Facts:</u>

Calories: 267

Carbs: 3 grams

Fat: 28 grams

Triple Layer Choconut Almond Butter Cups (Serves 12)

Ingredients:

Bottom Layer:

1/2 cup of Finely Chopped Cacao Paste

1/4 cup of Coconut Oil

1 teaspoon of Vanilla Powder

1/4 teaspoon of Ground Ceylon Cinnamon

2 to 3 drops of Pure Almond Extract

Middle Layer:

1/2 cup of All-Natural Almond Butter

1/4 cup of Coconut Oil

1/4 teaspoon of Ground Ceylon Cinnamon

Top Layer:

1/4 cup of Coconut Oil

1/2 cup of Creamy Coconut Butter

Whole Raw Almonds

Toasted Coconut Flakes

Directions:

1. Line your muffin pan with large parchment paper cups or silicone cups.

2. Melt 3/4 cup of coconut oil.

3. In your small-sized mixing bowl melt your cacao paste in the microwave in 20 to 30 second intervals and stir well for an equal amount of time between each melting session until there are no lumps left. Stir in 1/4 cup of the melted coconut oil, as well as your vanilla powder, cinnamon, and almond extract. Mix lightly until well combined.

4. Divide your melted chocolate equally between your 12 muffin cups and place in your refrigerator to set for approximately 5 minutes.

5. In a separate mixing bowl, add your almond butter, 1/4 cup of melted coconut oil, and ground cinnamon. Stir to combine, then pour your mixture over the set chocolate. Put your cups back into your refrigerator until that new layer has set. Should take approximately 5 to 10.

6. While your cups are in the refrigerator add 1/2 cup of creamy coconut butter to your bowl that you melted your coconut oil in (there should be 1/4 cup of oil left in it) and stir until well incorporated.

7. Gently spoon your mixture over the almond butter layer, then garnish each cup with a whole almond or a pinch of toasted coconut flakes.

8. Place in your refrigerator to finish setting, approximately 1 hour. These will keep for a few weeks if stored in the refrigerator in an airtight container.

9. Serve and Enjoy!

<u>Nutrition Facts:</u>

Calories: 298

Carbs: 6.5 grams

Fat: 29.5 grams

Matcha Coconut Fat Bombs (Serves 32)

<u>Ingredients:</u>

<u>Main:</u>

1/2 cup of Full Fat Coconut Milk (Refrigerated Overnight)

1 cup of Creamy Coconut Butter

1 cup of Firm Coconut Oil (Refrigerated Overnight)

1/2 teaspoon of Matcha Green Tea Powder

1/4 teaspoon of Himalayan Salt

1/4 teaspoon of Ground Ceylon Cinnamon

1 teaspoon of Pure Vanilla Extract

<u>Coating:</u>

1 cup of Finely Shredded Unsweetened Coconut

1 tablespoon of Matcha Green Tea Powder

<u>**Directions:**</u>

1. Add all the ingredients listed under "main" to a large-sized mixing bowl. Note that it's of utmost importance that your coconut oil be firm so send it to your refrigerator if you have to. Same goes for your coconut milk.

2. Mix on high speed with your hand mixer, until light and fluffy, then send to your refrigerator to firm up for about an hour.

3. While your mixture is firming up, combine your shredded coconut and matcha powder together in a large-sized mixing bowl. Set to the side.

4. Form the cold mixture into 32 small balls.

5. Roll your balls quickly between the palms of your hands to shape them, then drop each ball into your coconut / matcha mixture and roll them until completely coated.

6. Transfer your finished fat bombs to an airtight container and keep refrigerated for up to 2 weeks.

7. Serve and Enjoy!

<u>**Nutrition Facts:**</u>

Calories: 135

Carbs: 3 grams

Fat: 14 grams

Cardamom Orange Walnut Truffles (Serves 12)

Ingredients:

1 cup of Almond Butter

1/4 cup of Unsweetened Coconut Flakes or Shredded Coconut

1/4 cup of Coconut Oil

1/3 cup of Walnuts

2 teaspoons of Orange Zest

1/2 cup Unsweetened Shredded Coconut

Dash of Cardamom

Stevia

1 tablespoon of Cacao Powder (Optional)

Directions:

1. Place all of your ingredients except for your 1/2 cup of shredded coconut into a blender and blend well.

2. Place in your refrigerator or freezer to solidify.

3. Form small-sized balls from your mixture.

4. Roll your balls in the remaining 1/4 cup of shredded coconut.

5. Place in your refrigerator to set.

6. Serve and Enjoy!

Nutrition Facts:

Calories: 190

Net Carbs: 3 grams

Sugar-Free Maple Nut Fudge (Serves 24)

<u>Ingredients:</u>

8 ounce package of Mascarpone or Cream Cheese

1 cup of Organic Butter

1/4 cup of Swerve

1 teaspoon of Maple Extract

1 teaspoon of Stevia Glycerite

<u>Options:</u>

1/4 teaspoon of Ground Ginger

1 cup of Pecans or Walnuts

<u>Directions:</u>

1. In your small-sized saucepan, melt butter over a medium-high heat (heat until it turns brown, not black).

2. Add natural sweeteners until sweeteners dissolve and the mixture bubbles just a little.

3. Using a hand mixer on a low speed, add in extract and mascarpone.

4. Mix until well combined.

5. The mixture will not emulsify until it cools a little. I placed the mixture into my blender and combined until smooth which caused it to not separate. If you use a hand mixer, it keeps separating until cooled. So after it cools a bit, whip it together.

6. Stir in the nuts and ginger if using.

7. Place a piece of parchment in an 8 x 8 square baking pan. Pour your mixture into the pan lined with parchment. Refrigerate overnight, the mixture will thicken a lot. Remove from your pan, peel away parchment and cut into 1-inch cubes. Makes 24 servings.

8. Serve and Enjoy!

<u>Nutrition Facts:</u>

Calories: 110

Carbs: 19 grams

Sugar-Free Mounds Bars (Serves 24)

Ingredients:

1/3 cup of Organic Extra Virgin Coconut Oil

1/3 cup of Organic Coconut Milk

1/2 cup of Confectioner's Style Swerve

1 cup of Unsweetened Organic Finely Shredded Coconut

8 ounces of Dark Chocolate (85% Cacao)

Directions:

1. In your medium-sized saucepan, combine your coconut oil, coconut milk, and the sweetener.

2. Heat over a low heat, constantly mixing until the coconut oil has melted.

3. Add your shredded coconut and mix until well mixed.

4. Pour your mixture in a 9 x 5 inch silicone loaf pan. Press your mixture tightly and evenly to the bottom of your pan.

5. Refrigerate for 3 hours or until your mixture is solid.

6. Turn your pan upside down, gently press the bottom of your pan so that the solid mixture pops out.

7. Cut your mixture into bars.

8. Chop your chocolate into small-sized pieces, equal in size.

9. Melt 3 ounces of your chopped chocolate in a water bath or in a double boiler. Don't let the chocolate get too hot, heat it gently until it is melted, stirring occasionally.

10. Remove your melted chocolate from the heat. Add 1 ounce of chopped chocolate to your melted chocolate and mix occasionally to get a smooth mixture.

11. Dip your bars in the melted chocolate, put on parchment paper or on cooling rack and let the chocolate set.

12. When your chocolate coating is completely set, melt 3 ounces of the chopped chocolate in a water bath or in a double boiler. Don't let your chocolate get too hot, heat it gently until it is melted, stirring occasionally.

13. Remove the chocolate from your heat. Add the rest of your chopped chocolate (1 ounce) to your melted chocolate and mix occasionally to get a smooth mixture.

14. Dip your bars a second time in your melted chocolate, put on parchment paper or on cooling rack and allow your chocolate to set.

15. Serve and Enjoy!

Nutrition Facts:

Calories: 110

Net Carbs: 2.1 grams

Vanilla Fat Bombs (Serves 14)

Ingredients:

1 cup of Unsalted Macadamia Nuts

1/4 cup of Virgin Coconut Oil

1/4 cup of Butter

1 Vanilla Bean or 2 teaspoon of Sugar-Free Vanilla Extract

Optional:

10 to 15 drops of Stevia Extract

2 tablespoons of Swerve

Directions:

1. Place your macadamia nuts into your blender and pulse until smooth.

2. Mix with your softened butter and coconut oil (room temperature or melted in a water bath).

3. Add swerve, stevia, and vanilla bean.

4. Pour into your mini muffin forms or an ice cube tray. You should be able to fill each one about 1 1/2 tablespoons of your mixture to get 14 servings. Place in the refrigerator for approximately 30 minutes and let it solidify.

5. When done, keep refrigerated. Coconut oil and butter get soft at room temperature.

6. Serve and Enjoy!

Nutrition Facts:

Calories: 132

Net Carbs: 0.6 grams

Mint Fudge Fat Bombs

<u>Ingredients:</u>

1 1/2 cups of Coconut Oil

1 1/5 cups of Nut or Seed Butter

1/2 cup of Sweetener

1/2 cup of Dried Parsley Flakes

2 tablespoons of Vanilla

1 teaspoon of Peppermint Extract

1/4 tablespoon of Salt

Melted Chocolate

Directions:

1. Melt your coconut oil in a small-sized saucepan. Add your remaining ingredients to your blender, add your coconut oil and blend until smooth.

2. Pour into an 8x8 baking pan and freeze until solid.

3. Store in your refrigerator to prevent softening.

4. Serve and Enjoy!

Keto Fat Bomb Ice Cream (Serves 5)

<u>Ingredients:</u>

4 Yolks from Pastured Eggs

4 Whole Pastured Eggs

1/3 cup of Melted Coconut Oil

1/3 cup of Melted Cacao Butter

1/4 cup of MCT Oil

1/3 cup of Xylitol or 15 to 20 drops of Alcohol-Free Stevia

2 teaspoons of Vanilla Bean Powder

8 to 10 Ice Cubes

<u>Directions:</u>

1. Add all your ingredients but the ice cubes into the jug of your high powered blender. Blend on high for approximately 2 minutes, until creamy.

2. While your blender is still running, remove the top portion of the lid and drop in 1 ice cube at a time, allowing your blender to run about 10 seconds between each ice cube. The goal here is to dilute the mixture just a bit and make it cold so it will run through the ice cream maker easier.

3. Once all of your ice has been added, pour the cold mixture into your ice cream maker and churn on high for approximately 20 to 30 minutes, depending on your ice cream maker. If you do not have an ice cream maker, transfer the mixture to your 9x5 loaf pan and place in your freezer. Set your timer for approximately 30 minutes before taking it out to stir. Repeat for 2 to 3 hours, until desired consistency is met.

4. Serve immediately as soft-serve or scoop into a 9x5 loaf pan and freeze for approximately 45 minutes. Store covered in your freezer for up to a week.

5. Serve and Enjoy!

Peppermint Mocha Fat Bombs (Serves 16)

Ingredients:

3 tablespoons of Melted Coconut Oil

3/4 cup of Melted Coconut Butter

1/4 teaspoon of Peppermint Extract

3 tablespoons of Hemp Seeds

2 teaspoons of Instant Coffee Powder

2 tablespoons of Organic Cocoa Powder

5 to 8 drops of Liquid Stevia

Directions:

1. Mix together your melted coconut butter, 1 tablespoon of coconut oil, hemp seeds, and peppermint extract.

2. Pour into molds about 3/4 of the way.

3. Refrigerate until firm.

4. Stir together 2 tablespoons of melted coconut oil, cocoa powder, instant coffee, and stevia.

5. Drizzle on top of your fat bombs.

6. Refrigerate again until completely hardened.

7. Pop out of your molds and transfer to an airtight container.

8. Store in your refrigerator or freezer.

9. Serve and Enjoy!

Nutrition Facts:

Calories: 121

Carbs: 4 grams

Blackberry Coconut Fat Bombs (Serves 16)

Ingredients:

1 cup of Coconut Butter

1/2 cup of Fresh or Frozen Blackberries

1 cup of Coconut Oil

1/4 teaspoon of Vanilla Powder or 1/2 teaspoon of Vanilla Extract

1/2 teaspoon of Sweet Leaf Stevia Drops

1 tablespoon of Lemon Juice

Directions:

1. Place your coconut butter, coconut oil, and blackberries (if frozen) in a pot and heat over a medium heat until well combined.

2. In your food processor or small blender, add your coconut oil mix and remaining ingredients. Process until smooth. Separation may occur if coconut oil mixture is too hot. If using fresh berries, there is no need to cook them with the coconut oil and butter.

3. Spread out into a small-sized pan lined with parchment paper (I used a 6x6-inch container)

4. Refrigerate for one hour or until your mix has hardened.

5. Remove from your container and cut into squares.

6. Store covered in the refrigerator.

7. Serve and Enjoy!

<u>Nutrition Facts:</u>

Calories: 170

Carbs: 3 grams

Fat: 19 grams

White Chocolate Coconut Fudge (Serves 24)

Ingredients:

4 ounces of Cacao Butter

1/2 cup of Coconut Oil

15-ounce can of Coconut Milk

1 cup of Coconut Butter

1 teaspoon of Vanilla Extract

1/2 cup of Vanilla Protein Powder

1 teaspoon of Coconut Liquid Stevia

Pinch of Salt

Optional:

Unsweetened Coconut Flake

Directions:

1. Melt your cacao butter in your saucepan over a low heat.

2. Stir in your coconut milk, coconut oil, and coconut butter.

3. Continue to stir until completely smooth, no lumps.

4. Turn off your heat and whisk in protein powder, vanilla extract, stevia, and salt.

5. Pour your mixture into a parchment lined 8x8 pan.

6. Sprinkle with coconut flakes if desired.

7. Refrigerate for 4 hours or overnight.

8. Does not need to be kept refrigerated for storage.

9. Serve and Enjoy!

Nutrition Facts:

Calories: 175

Net Carbs: 1.2 grams

Daily Greens Fat Bomb Truffles (Serves 14)

<u>Ingredients:</u>

1 1/2 cups of Unsweetened Medium-Shredded Coconut

1/2 cup of Extra-Virgin Coconut Oil (At Room Temperature)

2 tablespoons of Greens+ O Powder (Vanilla Flavor)

<u>For Cacao Truffles add:</u>

1/4 cup of Cacao Powder

<u>Optional Toppings:</u>

Chia seeds

Hemp hearts

Unsweetened Medium-Shredded Coconut

Directions:

1. Line your small-sized baking sheet with parchment paper and set to the side. If you're going to add toppings to your truffles, place a couple of tablespoons of topping ingredients in separate small-sized bowls and set to the side.

2. Add your coconut and greens powder to your bowl of your stand mixer or food processor with dough blade, or a large-sized bowl and use a handheld mixer. Mix until your coconut is covered in greens, then add your coconut oil.

3. Mix until everything is well combined. The mixture should hold together.

4. Scoop dough, about 1 tablespoon at a time, into the palm of your hand. Roll lightly and place on your prepared baking sheet. Repeat with your remaining dough. Mixture should make 14 truffles.

5. Once completed, transfer your baking sheet to the refrigerator to cool for approximately 15 minutes.

6. Store in an air-tight container in your refrigerator for 5 days, or freezer for 2 months.

7. Serve and Enjoy!

Nutrition Facts:

Calories: 152

Net Carbs: 1.7 grams

White Chocolate Butter Pecan Fat Bombs (Serves 4)

Ingredients:

2 tablespoons of Coconut Oil

2 ounces of Cocoa Butter

2 tablespoons of Butter

2 tablespoons of Powdered Erythritol

1/2 cup of Chopped Pecans

1/4 teaspoon of Vanilla Extract

Pinch of Salt

Pinch of Stevia

Directions:

1. Melt your coconut oil, cocoa butter, and butter together in a small-sized pan until melted. Then turn your heat off.

2. Stir in 2 tablespoons of powdered erythritol into your butter mixture until well combined.

3. Add a pinch of salt to bring out the sweetness.

4. Add in a pinch of Stevia.

5. Add in your vanilla extract.

6. Into silicone cupcake molds or candy molds, add a few chopped pecans. I added about 3-4 pecans total to each mold, but this can be altered. If you don't have pecans, walnuts and hazelnuts work well.

7. Pour your white chocolate mix evenly into the molds over your nuts and place in the freezer immediately.

8. Freeze for about 30 minutes. You want them to be nice and cool when eating as they melt easily.

9. Serve and Enjoy!

<u>Nutrition Facts:</u>

Calories: 287

Carbs: 0.5 grams

Fat: 30 grams

Strawberry-Filled Coconut Fat Bombs (Serves 15)

Ingredients:

1/3 cup of Coconut Butter

1/2 tablespoon of Cocoa Powder

1/3 cup of Coconut Oil + 1 tablespoon

1 tablespoons of Unsweetened Shredded Coconut

1/3 cup of Diced Fresh Strawberries

8 to 10 drops of Liquid Stevia

Directions:

1. In your bain-marie, add the coconut butter, 1/3 cup of coconut oil, cocoa powder, and a few drops of liquid stevia. Heat until fully melted.

2. Meanwhile, in your small-sized frying pan, add your fresh strawberries and a few spoonfuls of water. Cook over a medium heat until soft. Mash with a fork. Add the berries to a blender with 1 tablespoon of melted coconut oil and a few more drops of liquid stevia. Blend until smooth.

3. Fill your molds with the melted coconut mixture. Add about 1 teaspoon of the strawberry mixture into each mold. Sprinkle with a few shreds of unsweetened coconut.

4. Place in your refrigerator until fully hardened; at least a couple of hours or overnight. Pop out of the molds and store in an air-tight container in the refrigerator.

5. Serve and Enjoy!

<u>Nutrition Facts:</u>

Calories: 106

Net Carbs: 1 gram

No-Bake Grasshopper Bars

Ingredients:

Mint Layer:

2 Hass Avocados

3/4 cup of Melted Coconut Oil

1/2 cup of Sweetener

4 cups of Organic Shredded Unsweetened Coconut

6 scoops of Stevia

3/8 teaspoon of Organic Peppermint Extract

3/4 teaspoon of Vanilla

1/4 teaspoon of Salt

Chocolate Layer:

1/2 cup of Coconut Oil

1/2 cup of Cocoa Powder

1/8 teaspoon of Salt

1/2 teaspoon of Vanilla

1/4 cup of Xylitol (blended preferred for smoothness)

Directions:

Mint Layer:

1. Lightly grease your 8x8 pan.

2. Place all your ingredients in high powered blender or a food processor. Process until blended. If you prefer the texture of coconut in the finished result, do not process completely.

3. Spread your mixture into prepared pan and place in freezer.

Chocolate Layer:

1. In a small-sized saucepan, melt your coconut oil and sweetener over a low heat.

2. Remove from your heat, add in the remaining ingredients, and stir to combine.

3. Pour over your chilled bottom layer. Return to your freezer until the chocolate layer is solid.

4. Cut into bars

5. Store covered in the refrigerator or freezer

6. Serve and Enjoy!

No Bake N'oatmeal Fudge Bars (Serves 16)

Ingredients:

N'oatmeal Crust & Topping:

1 cup of Coconut Oil

2 cups of Manitoba Harvest Hemp Hearts

1/4 cup of Birch-Sourced Xylitol

1/3 cup of Coconut Flour

1/2 cup of Unsweetened Fancy Shredded Coconut

1/2 teaspoon of Vanilla Extract

Dairy-free Fudge:

1/2 cup of Full-Fat Coconut Milk

10 ounces of Unsweetened Chocolate

10 drops of Alcohol-Free Stevia

Directions:

1. Line your 9x9 baking sheet with parchment paper draping over all sides for easy lifting.

2. Melt your coconut oil and xylitol in a large-sized saucepan over a medium heat. Whisk until xylitol granules have dissolved, about 2 minutes.

3. Add Manitoba Harvest Hemp Hearts, shredded coconut, coconut flour, and vanilla extract. Remove from the heat and combine with a spoon until your ingredients are well blended. Press half of your mixture into the bottom of the prepared pan. Reserve the other half for topping, set to the side.

4. Transfer the base to your refrigerator while you continue with the fudge layer.

5. Meanwhile, melt your chocolate and coconut milk in a small-sized heavy saucepan over a low heat, frequently stirring until smooth. Stir in your stevia and set to the side.

6. Take the base out of your fridge. Spoon the chocolate mixture over the crust in your pan, and spread evenly with a knife or the back of a spoon. If the bottom layer hasn't totally set, a couple of hemp hearts will lift up and mix in with the chocolate, so take your time.

7. Crumble the remaining hemp mixture over your chocolate layer, pressing in gently. Cover, and refrigerate 2 to 3 hours or overnight. Cut into 16 bars and enjoy!

8. Store in the refrigerator.

9. Serve and Enjoy!

Cinnamon Coffee Cake Collagen Fat Bombs (Serves 12)

Ingredients:

1/4 cup of Almond Butter

1/2 cup of Coconut Oil

1 tablespoon of Instant Coffee

1 packet of Vanilla Collagen

1 teaspoon of Cinnamon

Directions:

1. In your small-sized saucepan heat coconut oil and almond butter on low until melted.

2. You can also microwave the coconut oil for about 30 seconds until melted.

3. Stir together all your ingredients.

4. Pour into an 8x8 pan, mini muffin tins, or silicone/plastic candy molds. Freeze until firm.

5. Serve and Enjoy!

Blackberry Mascarpone Fat Bombs (Serves 9)

Ingredients:

1/2 cup of Blackberries (No Sugar Added)

1 cup of Coconut Oil

2 tablespoons of Mascarpone Cheese

1 cup of Coconut Butter

1/2 teaspoon of Lemon Juice

1/4 teaspoon of Vanilla Extract

1/2 teaspoon of Liquid Stevia

Directions:

1. Start by thawing blackberries in a small-sized bowl.

2. Once your blackberries are thawed place your mascarpone cheese, coconut oil, coconut butter, vanilla extract, lemon juice, and liquid stevia in a mixing bowl and mix on low until everything is combined well. The smoother the better.

3. Spoon into silicone cupcake liners.

4. Freeze for 30 minutes and keep refrigerated.

5. Serve and Enjoy!

<u>Nutrition Facts:</u>

Calories: 437

Net Carbs: 4 grams

Bulletproof Fat Bombs (Serves 20)

<u>Ingredients:</u>

1/4 cup of Butter (Grass-Fed or Extra Virgin Coconut Oil)

1 cup of Creamed Coconut Milk / Mascarpone Cheese or Full-Fat Cream Cheese

2 tablespoons of MCT Oil

1/4 cup of Erythritol or Swerve

2 tablespoons of Unsweetened Raw Cocoa Powder

1/2 cup of Strong Brewed Coffee or Caffeine-Free Chicory Coffee

10 to 15 drops of Liquid Stevia Extract

<u>Optional:</u>

1 teaspoon Rum Extract

Directions:

1. Place your softened creamed coconut milk (or mascarpone cheese), butter, MCT oil, and cocoa powder.

2. Add your powdered erythritol and stevia into a blender and pulse until smooth.

3. Pour in your prepared coffee (room temperature or lukewarm, not hot) and pulse again until smooth. Pour into your ice-cream maker and process. It may take anything between 30 to 60 minutes depending on your ice-cream maker. If you don't have an ice-cream maker pour your mixture directly into an ice tray or small muffin tin. You should be able to fit ~ 2 tablespoons per fat bomb or make smaller fat bombs. You can also use 1 to 2 teaspoons instant coffee powder instead of 1/2 cup of coffee. The mixture will be thicker and you won't need an ice-cream maker.

4. Spoon about 2 tablespoons of the ice-cream into an ice tray to make fat bomb shapes. Place in the freezer for 2 to 3 hours or until firm.

5. Serve and Enjoy!

Nutrition Facts:

Calories: 77

Net Carbs: 0.5 grams

French Toast Fat Bombs (Serves 24)

<u>Ingredients:</u>

1 stick of Softened Unsalted Butter

8 ounces of Softened Cream Cheese

1/3 cup of Maple-Flavored Syrup

1/2 cup of Almond Butter

1/3 cup of Golden Monk Fruit Sweetener

1 teaspoon of Maple Extract

1/2 teaspoon of Pure Vanilla Extract

<u>Directions:</u>

1. In your mixing bowl, using an electric mixer, mix all your ingredients until well-combined.

2. Freeze mixture for 30 minutes.

3. Remove mixing bowl from freezer and form mixture into balls or scoop and flatten into silicone mold. (If forming fat bombs into balls, line plate with parchment paper and set fat bombs atop parchment paper.)

4. Harden your fat bombs in freezer for 45 minutes.

5. Serve and Enjoy!

Nutrition Facts:

Calories: 100

Carbs: 6.9 grams

PBJ Fat Bombs (Serves 24)

Ingredients:

1/4 cup of Coconut Oil

2 cups of Frozen Raspberries

1 tablespoon of MCT Oil or Melted Coconut Oil

1/4 cup of Coconut Flour

3/4 cup of Peanut Butter

1/4 teaspoon of Powdered Stevia

Directions:

1. In your microwave-safe bowl, microwave frozen raspberries thawed, should take about 1 minute.

2. Combine all of your ingredients in a food processor and blend until well-combined.

3. Spoon your mixture into a silicone mold and freeze for 1 hour.

4. Remove from your freezer. Pop your fat bombs out of molds.

5. Serve and Enjoy!

<u>**Nutrition Facts:**</u>

Calories: 86

Carbs: 3.8 grams

Berries & Cream Fat Bombs (Serves 24)

Ingredients:

2 cups of Frozen Mixed Berries

6 tablespoons of Softened Butter

8 ounces of Softened Cream Cheese

2 tablespoons of Golden Monk Fruit Sweetener

1 teaspoon of Vanilla Extract

Directions:

1. In your microwave-safe bowl, microwave frozen berries until thawed, should take about 1 minute.

2. Combine all of your ingredients in a food processor and blend until well-combined.

3. Spoon your mixture into a silicone mold and freeze for 4 hours, preferably overnight.

4. Remove from your freezer. Pop your fat bombs out of molds.

5. Serve and Enjoy!

<u>Nutrition Facts:</u>

Calories: 61

Carbs: 2.9 grams

Blueberry Bliss Fat Bombs (Serves 30)

Ingredients:

2 cups of Raw Cashews (Boiled for 12 Minutes or Soaked for 2 Hours)

14 ounces of Frozen Blueberries

1 cup of Coconut Oil

1/2 cup of Coconut Butter

1/2 teaspoon of Stevia

Directions:

1. In your microwave-safe bowl, heat your blueberries for about 1 minute, until slightly warmed.

2. Combine all of your ingredients in your food processor and blend until well-combined.

3. Transfer your mixture to a medium-sized bowl and place in your freezer for approximately 30 minutes.

4. Remove your bowl from the freezer. Using your hands, form mixture into small-sized balls.

5. Place the balls on your pan or plate and return to your freezer for 30 minutes. I recommend putting them on a cookie sheet lined with parchment paper to avoid the bottoms sticking to your plate or pan.

6. Remove from your freezer.

7. Serve and Enjoy!

Nutrition Facts:

Calories: 161

Carbs: 6.1 grams

Cinnamon Roll Fat Bombs (Serves 24)

Ingredients:

Fat Bomb:

1/2 cup of Softened Butter

8 ounces of Softened Cream Cheese

1/2 cup of Golden Monk Fruit Sweetener

1/2 cup of Crunchy Almond Butter

1 teaspoon of Vanilla Extract

2 teaspoons of Cinnamon

Frosting:

1 1/2 ounces of Softened Cream Cheese

1 tablespoon of Heavy Whipping Cream

1/4 teaspoon of Vanilla Extract

2 teaspoons of Golden Monk Fruit Sweetener

<u>**Directions:**</u>

1. In your mixing bowl, using an electric mixer, mix all of your fat bomb ingredients until well-combined.

2. Refrigerate your mixture for approximately 30 minutes.

3. Line your plate with parchment paper.

4. Remove your mixing bowl from your refrigerator and form your mixture into balls. Set your fat bombs on top of the parchment-lined plate.

5. Harden the fat bombs in your freezer for approximately 45 minutes.

6. For your frosting, using an electric mixer in a small-sized bowl, mix together all of your ingredients until fully incorporated.

7. Remove your fat bombs from the freezer and frost.

8. Serve and Enjoy!

<u>**Nutrition Facts:**</u>

Calories: 103

Carbs: 6.5 grams

Butter Cream Fat Bombs (Serves 20)

Ingredients:

Fat Bomb:

4 ounces of Cream Cheese (Room Temperature)

4 ounces of Organic Grass-Fed Butter (Room Temperature)

1 teaspoon of Vanilla Extract

2 to 6 tablespoons of Swerve

Coating:

Lily's Dark Chocolate (Optional)

Almonds (Toasted & Roughly Chopped)

Directions:

1. Add your cream cheese, butter, and vanilla extract to your bowl. Cream your mixture with an electric mixer until evenly combined and super smooth. Start by adding 2 tablespoons of Swerve, adding more if necessary to taste.

2. Spoon into your molds and freeze until hardened.

3. If adding a chocolate layer, melt chocolate in a water bath (or the microwave). Allow it to come to room temperature before coating.

4. Remove butter cream fat bombs from your molds. Using a fork, dip into melted chocolate briefly and transfer to a parchment-lined plate. Repeat for a thicker coating.

5. Keep refrigerated or frozen.

6. Serve and Enjoy!

<u>Nutrition Facts:</u>

Calories: 61.25

Net Carbs: 0.25 grams

Cookies N' Cream Fat Bombs (Serves 6)

<u>**Ingredients:**</u>

<u>*Crumbs:*</u>

2 tablespoons of Cocoa Powder

2/3 cup of Almond Flour

2 to 3 tablespoons of Swerve

2 tablespoons of Melted Grass-Fed Butter or Ghee

1/2 teaspoon of Instant Coffee (Optional)

Pinch of Kosher Salt

<u>*Vanilla Cream:*</u>

2 teaspoons of Vanilla Extract

2/3 cup of Full Fat Coconut Milk

2 to 4 tablespoons of Xylitol Erythritol

2/3 cup of Heavy Whipping Cream

Pinch of Kosher Salt

Directions:

Crumbs:

1. Lightly toast your almond flour in a dry skillet or pan over a medium heat, until fully golden and fragrant (2 to 4 minutes).

2. Transfer your toasted almond flour to your small-sized bowl, and mix in your cocoa, sweetener, coffee (optional), and salt. Add in your butter and mix until thoroughly combined. Press about 1/3 of your mixture into cupcake liners or silicon molds and leave the remaining 2/3 as crumbs. Place both in your freezer while you make the vanilla cream.

Vanilla Cream:

1. Add your coconut milk, sweetener, and salt to your saucepan over a medium heat. Whisk until your sweetener has dissolved and the mixture is smooth. Transfer to your mixing bowl and allow it to cool completely.

2. Add your heavy whipping cream to a large chilled bowl and whip until soft peaks form. Mix in your vanilla extract and the cooled coconut and sweetener mixture. Once your mixture is smooth, fold in the frozen cookie crumble.

3. Pour your cookies 'n cream mixture into your prepared molds and freeze until solid. Allow to thaw for approximately 10 to 15 minutes before eating.

4. Serve and Enjoy!

Nutrition Facts:

Calories: 230

Carbs: 4 grams

Fat: 24 grams

Neapolitan Fat Bombs (Serves 24)

<u>Ingredients:</u>

1/2 cup of Butter

1/2 cup of Sour Cream

1/2 cup of Coconut Oil

2 tablespoons of Erythritol

1/2 cup of Cream Cheese

1 teaspoon of Vanilla Extract

2 tablespoons of Cocoa Powder

2 Medium Strawberries

25 drops of Liquid Stevia

Directions:

1. Combine all of your ingredients (except for cocoa powder, strawberries, and vanilla) in a bowl. Use an immersion blender to mix it together.

2. Separate your mixture between 3 bowls. Add your cocoa powder to one, vanilla to another, and strawberries to the last.

3. Pour your chocolate mixture into your fat bomb mold, then freeze for 30 minutes. Repeat with vanilla and strawberry layers.

4. Let freeze for at least 1 hour.

5. Serve and Enjoy!

Nutrition Facts:

Calories: 103

Net Carbs: 0.65 grams

Fall Season Fat Bombs

Ingredients:

2 tablespoons of Peanut Butter

1 tablespoon of Coconut Oil

1 tablespoon of Heavy Cream

1/4 teaspoon of Allspice

1 teaspoon of Cocoa Powder

4 to 5 drops of Liquid Sucralose

Directions:

1. Gather your ingredients together. Put 2 tablespoons of peanut butter into a cup or mold.

2. Add 1 tablespoon of coconut oil.

3. Pour in 1 tablespoon of heavy cream.

4. Add 1 teaspoon of cocoa powder and 1/4 teaspoon of allspice to your mixture.

5. Stir well, making sure to clean the edges down.

6. Freeze for about 2 hours.

7. Serve and Enjoy!

Nutrition Facts:

Calories: 185

Net Carbs: 3.25 grams

Vanilla Cheesecake Fat Bombs (Serves 18)

Ingredients:

9 ounces of Cream Cheese

2 ounces of Erythritol

2 Teaspoons of Vanilla Extract

1 cup of Heavy Cream

Directions:

1. Put your cream cheese, vanilla and erythritol into your kitchen aid and mix on low. Alternatively put into your bowl and mix with your hand mixer on a low speed for 2 minutes, pausing to scrape down the sides of your bowl with a spatula, so as to achieve a smooth consistent texture.

2. Add half of your heavy cream and mix for another 2 minutes. Allow your bowl to sit for 3 to 5 minutes as erythritol in its granulated form requires a little extra time to dissolve.

3. Add the other half of your heavy cream and mix on a medium speed for 3 minutes until your mixture is thick with firm peaks.

4. Gently spoon your mixture into a piping bag and pipe into mini cupcake liners. Set your fat bombs in your refrigerator for at least 1 hour.

5. Serve and Enjoy!

<u>Nutrition Facts:</u>

Calories: 88

Carbs: 1 gram

Red Velvet Fat Bombs (Serves 24)

Ingredients:

3 1/2 ounces of 90% Dark Chocolate (Sugar Free)

3 tablespoons of Natvia

3 1/2 ounces of Butter

4 1/2 ounces of Cream Cheese

1 teaspoon of Vanilla Extract

1/3 cup of Heavy Cream

4 drops of Red Food Coloring

Directions:

1. Melt your chocolate in a heatproof bowl over a small-sized pot of simmering water. Make sure that your bowl isn't touching the water, as this will cause your chocolate to burn.

2. While your chocolate is melting, mix together your remaining ingredients with a hand mixer on a medium speed for approximately 3 minutes. Ensure the mix is fully combined.

3. With your hand mixer on a low speed, slowly add your chocolate mixture to the other ingredients. Mix on a medium speed for 2 minutes.

4. Add your mixture to a piping bag and pipe the fat bomb mixture onto a lined tray. Set in your refrigerator for approximately 40 minutes.

5. Add your heavy cream to a whipping canister and apply to your fat bombs. (Make sure the cream and canister are cold for a better-whipped cream)

6. Serve and Enjoy!

<u>Nutrition Facts:</u>

Calories: 59

Net Carbs: 1 gram

Vanilla Strawberry Fudge Fat Bombs (Serves 32)

Ingredients:

Vanilla Layer:

8 ounces of Butter

8 ounces of Cream Cheese

2 tablespoons of Erythritol

1 tablespoon of Vanilla Extract

Strawberry Fudge Layer:

8 ounces of Butter

8 ounces of Cream Cheese

1 ounce of Low Carb Strawberry Protein Powder

Directions:

Vanilla Layer:

1. Line your baking tray with parchment paper and set to the side.

2. Place your softened cream cheese, softened butter, vanilla extract, and erythritol in your bowl and mix with your hand mixer on a low speed. Slowly build up to medium-high speed, until all your ingredients are well combined.

3. Pour your vanilla layer into the lined tray and smooth out as evenly as possible. Set in your refrigerator for approximately 30 minutes.

Strawberry Layer:

1. As you did with the vanilla layer, place your softened cream cheese, butter, and strawberry protein powder in your bowl. Mix on a low speed with your hand mixer. Slowly increase your speed to a medium-high until all of your ingredients are well combined.

2. Pour your strawberry layer on top of the vanilla layer, smooth it out and set in your refrigerator for 1 hour.

3. Cut your fudge into bite-sized pieces and keep it cool, as it will soften quickly in warm temperatures.

4. Serve and Enjoy!

<u>Nutrition Facts:</u>

Calories: 150

Carbs: 0.2 grams

Fat: 16 grams

Pina Colada Fat Bombs (Serves 16)

Ingredients:

2 teaspoons of Pineapple Essence

2 tablespoons of Gelatin

3 teaspoons of Erythritol

1/2 cup of Boiling Water

1 teaspoon of Rum Essence

1/2 cup of Coconut Cream

Directions:

1. Dissolve your gelatin and erythritol in your boiling water in a heatproof jug and add your pineapple essence.

2. Allow to cool for 5 minutes.

3. Add your coconut cream and rum extract and continue stirring for 2 minutes.

4. Pour into silicon molds and set for at least 1 hour, depending on the size of your mold.

5. Gently remove from your mold. Store in the refrigerator.

6. Serve and Enjoy!

<u>Nutrition Facts:</u>

Calories: 23

Carbs: 0.4 grams

Fat: 2 grams

Lemon & Poppyseed Fat Bombs (Serves 18)

Ingredients:

8 ounces of Softened Cream Cheese

1 tablespoon of Poppy Seeds

3 tablespoons of Erythritol

4 tablespoons of Sour Cream

2 tablespoons of Lemon Juice

1 Lemon (Zest Only)

Directions:

1. Place all of your ingredients in your bowl and using a hand mixer, mix on a low speed, when your ingredients are combined, mix on medium-high speed for approximately 3 minutes.

2. Gently spoon your mixture into mini cupcake cases or place into a piping bag and pipe into mini cupcakes cases. Refrigerate for at least 1 hour.

3. Serve and Enjoy!

Nutrition Facts:

Calories: 60

Carbs: 1 gram

Fat: 5 grams

Chocolate Kisses Fat Bombs (Serves 24)

Ingredients:

8 ounces of Softened Cream Cheese

1 teaspoon of Vanilla Essence

1/4 cup of Natvia Icing Mix

5 ounces of Sugar-Free Chocolate

7 ounces of Heavy Cream

Directions:

1. Add your chocolate to a small-sized heatproof bowl and place over a small-sized saucepan of simmering water, ensuring that your bowl doesn't touch the water.

2. Melt your chocolate completely and remove from the heat. Set to the side.

3. Place your softened cream cheese in your bowl, using your hand mixer, mix on a medium speed until smooth.

4. Add your Natvia Icing Mix and vanilla essence and mix on a low speed until combined.

5. Add your heavy cream and mix on a medium speed until smooth and beginning to thicken.

6. Pour in your melted chocolate and mix on a medium speed, until all your ingredients are completely combined and the mixture is firm enough to pipe.

7. Add your mixture to a piping bag with a star nozzle. Pipe evenly into mini cupcake papers. Fill 24 cupcake papers, depending on your piping skills, you may get more or less.

8. Cover the kisses and set in your refrigerator for approximately 3 hours, or overnight.

9. They can be stored, covered in your refrigerator for up to 1 week, or frozen for up to 3 months.

10. Serve and Enjoy!

<u>Nutrition Facts:</u>

Calories: 80

Carbs: 4 grams

Fat: 6 grams

Chapter Three: Savory Keto Fat Bomb Recipes

In this section, I will show you 25+ savory ketogenic fat bomb recipes you can cook for yourself. These are keto fat bombs are geared towards people wanting to satisfy their savory side. These recipes are easy to prepare no matter what your level in the kitchen. These delicious treats will help keep you on track with your ketogenic diet.

Pizza Fat Bombs (Serves 6)

Ingredients:

4 ounces of Cream Cheese

8 Pitted Black Olives

14 slices of Pepperoni

2 tablespoons of Chopped Fresh Basil

2 tablespoons of Sun-Dried Tomato Pesto

Salt

Pepper

Directions:

1. Dice your pepperoni and olives into small-sized pieces.

2. Mix together your cream cheese, basil, and tomato pesto.

3. Add your olives and pepperoni into your cream cheese and mix again.

4. Form into balls, then garnish with pepperoni, olive, and basil.

5. Serve and Enjoy!

Nutrition Facts:

Calories: 101

Net Carbs: 1.7 grams

Salmon Fat Bombs (Serves 6)

Ingredients:

1/3 cup of Grass-Fed Butter

1/2 cup of Full-Fat Cream Cheese

1 tablespoon of Fresh Lemon Juice

1/2 package of Smoked Salmon or Smoked Mackerel

1 to 2 tablespoons of Freshly Chopped Dill (Skip if Using Mackerel)

Pinch of Salt

Directions:

1. Place your cream cheese, butter, and smoked salmon into a food processor.

2. Add fresh lemon juice and dill and pulse until smooth. I'm using your mixer with a food processor attachment.

3. Line a tray with parchment paper and create small-sized fat bombs using about 2 1/2 tablespoons of the mixture per piece. Garnish with more dill and place in your refrigerator for 1 to 2 hours or until firm.

4. Alternatively, simply spoon the mixture into an airtight container. Eat immediately or store in your refrigerator for up to a week. When ready to be served, just spoon out about 2 1/2 tablespoons per serving. Eat on top of crunchy lettuce leaves.

5. Serve and Enjoy!

Nutrition Facts:

Calories: 147

Net Carbs: 0.7 grams

Salmon Breakfast Bombs (Serves 2)

Ingredients:

Breakfast Bombs:

4 ounces of Sliced Smoked Salmon

2 Large Eggs

2 tablespoons of Chopped Fresh Chives

1/2 tablespoon of Salted Butter

Salt

Pepper

Hollandaise Sauce:

2 tablespoons of Salted Butter

1/4 teaspoon of Dijon Mustard

1 Large Egg Yolk (Separated From the White)

1/2 tablespoon of Water

2 teaspoons of Lemon Juice (Freshly Squeezed)

Salt

Directions:

1. Ensure you have all of your ingredients for hollandaise ready and sitting at room temperature.

2. Grab a small-sized pot and fill with water then put on your stove to boil. Once your water is boiling add your 2 whole eggs and let them boil for 10 to 12 minutes. You want your eggs to be hard boiled as we will be adding hollandaise to these.

3. While you are waiting for your eggs to boil, take your salmon slices and finely dice. Make sure they are separated once cut.

4. Preheat a pan over a high-heat and add your 2 teaspoons of butter. Once your butter has heated up, take approximately half of the cut up salmon and add into your pan then crisp into little crunchy pieces. Set to the side.

5. Once your eggs have boiled for approximately 10 to 12 minutes run your eggs and pot under cold water and allow your eggs to cool before peeling.

6. When your eggs have cooled, place them in a dish and use your fork to finely mash the egg.

7. After you have your eggs and salmon prepared you can make a start on your hollandaise. Don't try and do this at the same time as it will need your full attention to avoid clumps and splitting.

8. Take a pot and fill with a cup or two of water and place on your stove to simmer. Melt your 2 tablespoons of butter in the microwave for 30 to 60 seconds. You want your butter to be melted but not hot. Set to the side. In a large-sized heat-safe bowl whisk your egg yolk, lemon juice, dijon mustard and a pinch of salt together until you see air bubbles. Place your bowl with egg mixture over your pot with the simmering water to create a double boiler. Make sure that your water does not touch the bottom of the bowl.

9. Use a medium heat and continuously whisk your mixture until it starts to thicken.

10. Once the mixture starts thickening, slowly pour in your melted butter while stirring with a whisk. Ensure you keep stirring the entire time to avoid clumps. Once all of your butter is added, place your bowl back onto the pot to thicken further.

11. When your sauce has fully thickened you can remove it and set to the side. If your sauce is too thick add a tiny bit of water to thin, but remember you want a thick consistency.

12. Allow your hollandaise to cool to room temperature. You don't want to cook the salmon when you add the hollandaise, so it is crucial this is cool.

13. Take the raw salmon. hollandaise, half the chives, and mix well with your mashed egg. This should form a firm mixture.

14. Once combined, split your mixture into four pieces and roll into balls.

15. Mix your remaining chives and the crispy salmon together and roll your bombs in this to coat.

16. Serve and Enjoy!

<u>Nutrition Facts:</u>

Calories: 295

Net Carbs: 1 gram

Salmon and Dill Fat Bombs (Serves 12)

<u>Ingredients:</u>

1 cup of Cream Cheese

1/2 package of Smoked Salmon

2/3 cup of Butter

Lemon Juice (To Taste)

Salt (To Taste)

Dill (To Taste)

<u>Directions:</u>

1. Add all of your ingredients into a food processor and blend.

2. Create small-sized balls with your mixture and pop in your refrigerator.

3. Serve and Enjoy!

<u>Nutrition Facts:</u>

Calories: 174

Bacon Guacamole Deviled Eggs (Serves 6)

Ingredients:

4 strips of Thick Cut Bacon (Cooked Crisp & Crumbled)

6 Large Eggs

1 Large Avocado

1 tablespoon of Minced Garlic

2 tablespoons of Salsa

1 tablespoon of Dried Onion Flakes

1 tablespoon of Lime Juice

1/2 teaspoon of Garlic Salt

Pinch Cayenne Pepper

<u>**Directions:**</u>

1. Hard boil your eggs. Place your eggs in a large-sized saucepan with cold water. Add enough water that your eggs are fully submerged. Over a high heat bring your water to a rolling boil. Once your water is boiling, remove the pan from the heat, cover and allow it to sit for 12 minutes.

2. In your large-size mixing bowl, fork mash the avocado. Peel your eggs and slice in half lengthwise. Scrape the yolks out into your mixing bowl. To your bowl, add your bacon, salsa, garlic, lime juice, onion flakes, garlic salt, and cayenne pepper. Mix until all your ingredients are well incorporated.

3. Put your mixture into a plastic bag. Squeeze your mixture to one corner of the bag and snip off the corner of the bag. Use this to pipe the mixture into your eggs.

4. Serve and Enjoy!

<u>**Nutrition Facts:**</u>

Calories: 140

Net Carbs: 2.8 grams

Bacon Wrapped Mozzarella Sticks (Serves 2)

Ingredients:

1 Frigo Cheese Heads Mozzarella Cheese Stick (Cut In Half)

2 slices of Bacon

Coconut Oil (For Frying)

Low-Sugar Pizza Sauce (Optional)

Toothpicks

Directions:

1. Preheat your coconut oil in your deep fryer to 350 degrees.

2. Wrap your cut in half cheese sticks with your bacon, overlapping as you go just a bit so the bacon stays on. At the end of the wrapping, secure with your toothpick.

3. Drop your bacon wrapped cheese in your hot oil and cook until your bacon is brown and crispy, should take approximately 2 to 3 minutes.

4. Remove to a paper towel to cool for a few minutes. Remove the toothpick and serve with your favorite low-sugar dipping sauce.

5. Enjoy!

Nutrition Facts:

Calories: 103

Net Carbs: 1 gram

Bacon & Guacamole Fat Bombs (Serves 6)

<u>Ingredients:</u>

1/2 Large Avocado

4 Large Slices of Bacon

1/4 cup of Butter or Ghee (Softened at Room Temperature)

2 cloves of Crushed Garlic

1/2 Small Diced White Onion

1 Small Finely Chopped Chili Pepper

1 tablespoon of Fresh Lime Juice

1 to 2 tablespoons of Freshly Chopped Cilantro

1/4 teaspoon of Salt

Freshly Ground Black Pepper

Directions:

1. Preheat your oven to 375 degrees. Line your baking tray with parchment paper. Lay your bacon strips out flat on your parchment paper, leaving space so they don't overlap. Place your tray in the oven and cook for approximately 10 to 15 minutes until golden brown. The time depends on the thickness of your bacon slices. When done, remove from your oven and set to the side to cool down.

2. Halve, deseed and peel your avocado. Place your avocado, crushed garlic, butter, chili pepper, lime juice, and cilantro into your bowl and season with salt and pepper.

3. Mash using a potato masher or a fork until well combined. Add your diced onion and mix well.

4. Pour in your bacon grease from the tray where you baked the bacon and mix well. Cover with your foil and place in the refrigerator for 20 to 30 minutes.

5. Crumble your bacon into small-sized pieces and prepare for "breading." Remove your guacamole mixture from the refrigerator and start creating 6 balls. You can use a spoon or an ice-cream scooper. Roll each ball in your bacon crumbles and place on a tray that will fit in the refrigerator.

6. Serve and Enjoy!

Nutrition Facts:

Calories: 156

Net Carbs: 1.4 grams

Bacon, Pistachio, and Braunshweiger Truffles (Serves 12)

Ingredients:

8 ounces Braunshweiger Liverwurst (Room Temperature)

8 slices of Bacon (Cooked Crisp & Chopped Finely)

1/4 cup of Chopped Pistachio Kernels

1 teaspoon of Dijon Mustard

6 ounces of Softened Cream Cheese

Directions:

1. Combine your Braunshweiger and pistachios in a small-sized food processor and pulse until combined.

2. In a separate small-sized bowl, whip your softened cream cheese and mustard together until smooth.

3. Roll your Braunshweiger into 12 small balls.

4. Then take each ball and form about a 1/4 inch thick layer of cream cheese with your fingers.

5. Once you have done all of them, chill for approximately 30 minutes.

6. Roll each ball in the finely chopped bacon and place on a serving dish.

7. Serve and Enjoy!

<u>Nutrition Facts:</u>

Calories: 145

Net Carbs: 1.5 grams

Egg & Bacon Fat Bombs (Serves 6)

Ingredients:

2 Large Eggs

4 Large Slices of Bacon

2 tablespoons of Mayonnaise

1/4 cup of Softened Butter or Ghee

1/4 teaspoon of Salt

Freshly Ground Black Pepper

Directions:

1. Preheat your oven to 375 degrees. Line your baking tray with parchment paper. Lay your bacon strips out flat on the parchment paper, leaving space so they don't overlap. Place your tray in the oven and cook for approximately 10 to 15 minutes until golden brown. The time depends on the thickness of the bacon slices. When done, remove from your oven and set to the side to cool down.

2. Boil your eggs. Fill a small-sized saucepan with water up to three quarters. Add a good pinch of salt. This will prevent your eggs from cracking. Bring to a boil. Using a spoon or hand, dip each egg in and out of your boiling water - be careful not to get burnt. This will prevent your egg from cracking as the temperature change won't be so dramatic. To get your eggs hard-boiled, you need approximately 10 minutes. This timing works for large eggs. When done, remove from your heat and place in a bowl filled with cold water. When chilled, peel off the shells.

3. Cut the butter into small-sized pieces and add your peeled and quartered eggs. Mash with a fork.

4. Add your mayonnaise, season with pepper and salt and mix together well. Pour in your bacon grease and combine well. Place in your refrigerator for approximately 20 to 30 minutes or until it's solid and easy to form fat bombs.

5. Crumble your bacon into small-sized pieces and prepare for "breading." Remove your egg mixture from the fridge and start creating 6 balls. You can use a spoon or an ice-cream scooper. Roll each ball in the bacon crumbles and place on a tray that will fit in the refrigerator.

6. Serve and Enjoy!

<u>Nutrition Facts:</u>

Calories: 185

Net Carbs: 0.2 grams

Buffalo Chicken Deviled Eggs (Serves 6)

Ingredients:

6 ounces of Chicken (Cooked & Chopped)

6 Large Eggs (Hard Boiled)

1/4 Small Onion

1/4 cup of Franks Buffalo Wing Sauce

1/4 cup of Blue Cheese Crumbles

2 tablespoons of Blue Cheese Dressing

Chopped Small Rib Celery

Directions:

1. While your eggs are boiling, chop up your chicken and the celery.

2. Peel your eggs and slice in half lengthwise. Scrape your yolks out into a large-sized mixing bowl. To your bowl add the rest of the ingredients except for your onion. Grate the onion over your bowl. The juice from your onion will add a lot of flavor to your mixture.

3. Mix all your ingredients together. Put your mixture into a Ziploc bag. Squeeze the mixture to one corner of the bag and snip off the corner of your bag. Use this to pipe the mixture into your eggs.

4. Serve and Enjoy!

Nutrition Facts:

Calories: 111

Net Carbs: 1.3 grams

Bacon-Wrapped Mini Meatloaves (Serves 4)

Ingredients:

1 pound of Ground Beef

1/4 cup of Coconut Milk

1/2 pound of Bacon (Cut In Small Chunks)

8 strips of Bacon

1/3 cup of Minced Fresh Chives

2 Minced Garlic Cloves

Chopped Fresh Parsley

Freshly Ground Black Pepper

Directions:

1. Preheat your oven to 400 F.

2. In a large-sized bowl, combine your ground beef, bacon chunks, garlic, chives, and your coconut milk. Mix well until all of your ingredients hold together.

3. Season your mixture with freshly ground black pepper. No need to add salt to your mixture since the bacon is already salty enough.

4. Take a medium size muffin tin and place a slice of bacon around the sides of each hole.

5. Fill these same eight holes with your beef mixture.

6. Place in your oven and cook for approximately 30 minutes.

7. Once ready and cool enough to handle, remove your mini meatloaves from the muffin tin and add fresh parsley sprinkled on top.

8. Serve and Enjoy!

Nutrition Facts:

Carbs: 2 grams

Fat: 51 grams

Jalapeno Popper Deviled Eggs w/ Bacon

Ingredients:

6 Large Eggs

6 slices of Bacon (Cooked Crisp & Crumbled)

16 Sliced Pickled Jalapenos (Divided)

2 ounces of Softened Cream Cheese

4 to 6 tablespoons of Mayonnaise

1/4 teaspoon of Smoked Paprika

Directions:

1. Hard boil your eggs. Place your eggs in a large-sized saucepan with cold water. Add enough water that your eggs are fully submerged. Over a high heat bring your water to a rolling boil. Once your water has come to a boil, remove the pan from the heat, cover and allow it to sit for approximately 12 minutes.

2. Chop 4 of the jalapeno slices and set to the side.

3. Peel your eggs and slice in half lengthwise. Remove the yolks and fork mash them in your medium mixing bowl. To your bowl, add bacon, cream cheese, mayonnaise, and chopped jalapenos. Mix until all of your ingredients are well incorporated.

4. Spoon your mixture into a plastic bag or pastry bag. Squeeze the mixture to one corner of your bag and snip off the corner. Use this to pipe the filling into your egg halves.

5. Top each egg with a jalapeno slice. Sprinkle your paprika over top of the eggs.

6. Serve and Enjoy!

Cheesy Jalapeno Fat Bombs (Serves 6)

Ingredients:

3 1/2 ounces of Full-Fat Cream Cheese (Room Temperature)

4 slices of No-Sugar Bacon

1/4 cup of Unsalted Butter or Ghee (Room Temperature)

2 Jalapeño Peppers (Halved, Seeded, & Finely Chopped

1/4 cup of Grated Gruyère Cheese or Cheddar Cheese

Directions:

1. In your bowl, mash together your cream cheese and butter, or process in a food processor until smooth.

2. Preheat your oven to 325 degrees.

3. Line your rimmed baking sheet with parchment paper. Be sure to use a rimmed sheet to contain the bacon fat.

4. Lay your bacon slices flat on the parchment, leaving enough space between so they don't overlap.

5. Place your sheet in the preheated oven and cook for approximately 25 to 30 minutes, or until crispy. The exact amount of cooking time depends on the thickness of bacon slices.

6. Remove from your oven and set to the side to cool. When cool enough to handle, crumble your bacon into a bowl and set to the side.

7. To your cream cheese and butter mixture, add the Gruyère or Cheddar cheese, jalapeños, and bacon grease. Mix well to combine. Refrigerate for approximately 30 minutes to 1 hour, or until set.

8. Divide your mixture into 6 fat bombs and place them on a parchment-lined plate. If serving immediately, roll them in your crumbled bacon until well coated. If serving later, refrigerate without the bacon coating in an airtight container for up to 1 week. Roll the fat bombs in freshly cooked or reheated bacon crumbs just before serving.

9. Serve and Enjoy!

<u>Nutrition Facts:</u>

Calories: 208

Net Carbs: 0.7 grams

Savory Mediterranean Fat Bombs (Serves 5)

<u>Ingredients:</u>

1/4 cup of Softened Butter or Ghee

1/2 cup of Cream Cheese (Full-Fat)

2 to 3 tablespoons of Freshly Chopped Herbs (Basil, Thyme, & Oregano)

4 pieces of Drained Sun-Dried Tomatoes

4 Pitted Olives

5 tablespoons of Grated Parmesan Cheese

2 cloves of Crushed Garlic

1/4 teaspoon of Salt

Freshly Ground Black Pepper

Directions:

1. Cut your butter into small-sized pieces and place in your bowl with the cream cheese. Leave it on a kitchen counter for approximately 20 to 30 minutes to soften. Mash with your fork and mix until well combined. Add your chopped sun-dried tomatoes and chopped olives.

2. Add your freshly chopped herbs, crushed garlic, and season with salt and pepper. Mix well and place in your refrigerator for approximately 20 to 30 minutes to solidify.

3. Remove your cheese mixture from the refrigerator and start creating 5 balls. You can use a spoon or an ice-cream scooper. Roll each ball in the grated Parmesan cheese and place on your plate. Eat immediately or store in your refrigerator in an airtight container for up to a week.

4. Serve and Enjoy!

Nutrition Facts:

Calories: 165

Net Carbs: 1.7 grams

Keto Butter Burgers Fat Bombs (Serves 12)

Ingredients:

1 pound of Ground Beef (85% Lean)

2 ounces of Cheese

3 tablespoons of Butter

Pepper

Salt

Garlic Powder (Optional)

Onion Powder (Optional)

Directions:

1. Preheat your oven to 375 degrees.

2. In a medium-sized bowl, combine your ground beef with your desired amount of salt and pepper. Optionally, add your onion powder and/or garlic powder.

3. Press a small amount of beef (about 1 tablespoon) into the bottom of your non-stick, 12-slot muffin pan so the bottom is fully covered.

4. Add a pat of butter to the top of each piece of beef.

5. Add beef to the top. Press to flatten.

6. Add a small piece of cheese to your beef.

7. Add a final layer of beef. Press to flatten.

8. Place your muffin pan in the oven and bake for approximately 10 minutes.

9. When the baking is complete, turn off your oven and crack the oven door for a few minutes to release the heat (if using a silicone muffin pan, wait approximately 10 minutes).

10. Using a fork, remove each butter burger from your pan and place on your plate.

11. There will be a beef fat/butter combo remaining in your muffin pan. Save this and use it to drizzle on your butter burgers.

12. Serve and Enjoy!

Nutrition Facts:

Calories: 125

Fat: 10 grams

Savory Sesame Fat Bombs (Serves 4)

Ingredients:

4 ounces of Butter (Room Temperature)

1 teaspoon of Sea Salt

2 tablespoons of Sesame Oil

2 teaspoons of Toasted Sesame Seeds

1/4 teaspoon of Chili Flakes

Directions:

1. Start by adding sesame seeds to a dry, hot pan and roast them for a couple of minutes while stirring the entire time; be careful not to burn them. Once they are golden brown and start popping, they are done. Transfer immediately to a plate or shallow bowl and set to the side.

2. Mix your butter, sesame oil, chili flakes, and salt in your small-sized bowl. Place in the refrigerator for approximately 15 minutes or more.

3. Shape your butter mixture into balls the size of walnuts, approximately half an ounce. Roll each ball in the toasted sesame seeds. Store in your refrigerator or freezer.

4. Serve and Enjoy!

Sausage Balls Fat Bombs (Serves 23)

Ingredients:

1 pound of Breakfast Sausage

1 cup of Almond Flour

1 Large Egg

1/4 cup of Grated Parmesan

8 ounces of Cheddar Cheese

2 teaspoons of Baking Powder

1 tablespoon of Butter (or Coconut Oil)

1/4 teaspoon of Salt

Directions:

1. Preheat oven to 350 degrees.

2. Add your eggs and spices to your bowl and beat until well combined.

3. Add all other ingredients to your egg mixture.

4. Using your cookie scoop and your hands roll sausage mixture into 20 to 25 sausage balls.

5. Place sausage balls on a cookie sheet.

6. Bake for approximately 16 to 20 minutes.

7. Store in a sandwich bag or covered bowl in your refrigerator.

8. Serve and Enjoy!

Nutrition Facts:

Calories: 124

Carbs: 1 gram

Bacon Burger Bombs (Serves 12)

Ingredients:

12 slices of Bacon

12 Rounds Raw Sausage Patties (1-Ounce Each)

12 Cubes Smoked Cheddar Cheese (1-Inch)

Cumin (To Taste)

Onion Powder (To Taste)

Pepper (To Taste)

Salt (To Taste)

Directions:

1. Preheat your oven to 350 degrees. Lay out your sausage rounds on a cookie sheet lined with your parchment paper.

2. Dust your sausage with cumin, onion powder, pepper, and salt.

3. Place a piece of cheese in the middle of your sausage rounds.

4. Form a ball around your cheese with the sausage. Roll it in your hands to make a good circle shape.

5. Wrap your bacon around your sausage balls.

6. Bake at 350 degrees for an hour.

7. Serve and Enjoy!

<u>Nutrition Facts:</u>

Calories: 250

Net Carbs: 1.4 grams

Sausage Ball Puffs (Serves 36)

Ingredients:

1 pound of Breakfast Sausage (Drained & Browned)

4 Eggs

4 1/2 tablespoons of Melted Butter & Cooled)

2 tablespoons of Full Fat Sour Cream

1/3 cup of Coconut Flour

2 cups of Sharp Shredded Cheddar Cheese

1/4 teaspoon of Baking Powder

1/4 teaspoon of Salt

Directions:

1. Preheat your oven to 375 degrees and grease your cookie sheet.

2. Combine your melted butter (I cool mine by popping the bowl in the refrigerator for 5 minutes), eggs, salt, and sour cream then whisk together.

3. Add your coconut flour and baking powder to your mixture and stir until combined.

4. Add your drained browned sausage.

5. Stir in your cheese.

6. Drop batter by tightly packed spoonfuls on your greased cookie sheet.

7. Bake for approximately 15 to 18 minutes or until tops are slightly brown.

8. Serve and Enjoy!

Nutrition Facts:

Calories: 89

Carbs: 0.6 grams

Fat: 7 grams

Cheesy Bacon Fat Bombs (Serves 20)

Ingredients:

8 ounces of Mozzarella Cheese

10 slices of Bacon

4 tablespoons of Melted Butter

4 tablespoons of Almond Flour

1 Large Egg

3 tablespoons of Psyllium Husk Powder

1/4 teaspoon of Black Pepper

1/4 teaspoon of Salt

1/8 teaspoon of Onion Powder

1/8 teaspoon of Garlic Powder

1 cup of Oil (For Frying)

<u>**Directions:**</u>

1. Microwave half of your cheese for 45 to 60 seconds or until it is melted.

2. Microwave butter for 15 to 20 seconds until fully melted, then pour butter into your cheese and egg.

3. Mix together and add psyllium husk, almond flour, and spices. Mix together again and pour dough out onto a silpat.

4. Pretty dough and roll out into a rectangle. Fill your rectangle with the rest of your cheese and fold in half (horizontally), then in half again (vertically).

5. Crimp edges and re-form into a rectangle. Cut out 20 squares from this.

6. Wrap each piece of your dough in half of a piece of bacon tightly, using toothpicks to secure the bacon.

7. Heat oven to 375 degrees, then fry each cheesy bacon bomb for 1 to 3 minutes each.

8. Remove from your oil and allow it to cool on your paper towels.

9. Serve and Enjoy!

Nutrition Facts:

Calories: 93

Net Carbs: 0.65 grams

Sausage & Cream Cheese Fat Bombs (Serves 8)

Ingredients:

1 pound of Uncooked Hot Sausage

1 cup of Shredded Cheddar Cheese

2 cups of Bisquick Baking Mix

8-ounce block of Cream Cheese

Directions:

1. Preheat your oven to 350 degrees.

2. Line your baking sheets with parchment paper.

3. In the bowl of a stand mixer, mix together your sausage and cream cheese.

4. Add in your baking mix and stir until combined.

5. Add in your cheese.

6. Stir until well combined.

7. Scoop up meat mixture and form into 1-inch balls and place on your baking sheet.

8. Once you have them all on the baking sheet, just go back and roll them around in your hands to make them a bit more smooth on the outside. Pop your baking sheet in the refrigerator for approximately 10 minutes.

9. Once they are chilled, bake for approximately 25 minutes.

10. Serve and Enjoy!

<u>Nutrition Facts:</u>

Calories: 357

Carbs: 19 grams

Breakfast Bacon Fat Bombs (Serves 6)

Ingredients:

1 Large Hardboiled Egg

6 Cooked Bacon Slices

1/4 Avocado

6 Cooked Bacon Slices

4 tablespoons of Unsalted or Clarified Butter

1 tablespoon of Mayonnaise

2 tablespoons of Bacon Grease

1 Serrano Pepper (Seeded & Diced)

1 tablespoon of Chopped Cilantro

1/4 Juice of Lime

Kosher Salt (To Taste)

Cracked Pepper (To Taste)

Directions:

1. In your large-sized bowl, combine your hardboiled egg, butter, avocado, serrano pepper, mayonnaise, and cilantro. Mash into a smooth paste with your fork or potato masher. Season with salt and pepper, then add your lime juice and stir.

2. Prepare your bacon in your favorite fashion until crispy, reserving 2 tablespoons of bacon grease. Add your bacon grease to the fat bomb mixture and stir gently. Cover and place in your refrigerator for 30 minutes, or until the mixture has cooled and can form solid balls. Crumble your bacon into small bits in a small-sized bowl.

3. Using your spoon, scoop out 6 even-sized amounts of your fat bomb mixture and form into balls. Add the balls to your bacon bits and roll around until completely covered.

4. Serve and Enjoy!

Baked Brie & Pecan Prosciutto Fat Bombs (Serves 1)

Ingredients:

1/2 ounce of Prosciutto

1/8 teaspoon of Black Pepper

6 Pecan Halves

1-ounce Full-Fat Brie Cheese

Directions:

1. Preheat oven to 350 degrees. Use your muffin tin, whose muffin holes are about 2.5 inch wide and 1.5 inch deep.

2. Take the prosciutto and fold it in half so it becomes almost square.

3. Place it in a hole of the muffin tin to line it completely.

4. Chop your Brie in little cubes, leaving the white skin on. Place your Brie in the prosciutto-lined cup.

5. Stick your pecan halves in amongst the Brie.

6. Bake for approximately 12 minutes, until your Brie is melted and prosciutto is cooked.

7. Allow it to cool for approximately 10 minutes before removing from the muffin pan.

8. Serve and Enjoy!

<u>**Nutrition Facts:**</u>

Calories: 183

Net Carbs: 0.4 grams

Pepperoni Pizza Fat Bombs (Serves 6)

Ingredients:

3 1/2 ounces of Cream Cheese (Room Temperature)

1 clove of Minced Garlic

12 Pepperoni Slices

1/2 Finely Chopped Small Red Pepper

1/3 cup of Grated Parmesan Cheese

1/4 cup of Unsalted Butter (Room Temperature)

1/4 cup of Grated Mozzarella Cheese

2 tablespoons of Chopped Fresh Herbs (Basil, Oregano, or Thyme)

1/8 teaspoon of Chili Powder

Pinch of Salt

Directions:

1. In your bowl, mash together your cream cheese and the butter with a fork, or process in a food processor until smooth.

2. In a large-sized skillet, set over a medium heat, cook your pepperoni slices on both sides until crispy. Transfer to your plate to cool.

3. Add the garlic and red pepper to the pepperoni juices in the skillet and cook for a few minutes over a medium heat until fragrant. Remove from the heat and cool slightly. Add to your cream cheese and butter mixture and mix well with an electric beater or a hand whisk.

4. Add your grated mozzarella cheese, salt, herbs, and chili powder. Mix well again. Refrigerate for 20 to 30 minutes, or until set.

5. Using a large spoon or an ice cream scoop, divide the mixture into 6 balls. Roll each ball in your Parmesan cheese and place on top of 2 slices of crisped pepperoni. Refrigerate in an airtight container for up to 5 days.

6. Serve and Enjoy!

Bacon Wrapped Chicken Bombs (Serves 6)

<u>Ingredients:</u>

2 pounds of Boneless, Skinless Chicken Breasts

4 ounces of Softened Cream Cheese

10 ounces of Frozen Spinach

12 slices of Bacon

1/2 cup of Full-Fat Ricotta

Pepper

Salt

<u>Directions:</u>

1. Thaw your spinach out and wring as much water out of it as possible. Preheat your oven to 375 degrees.

2. Mix your spinach with the cream cheese and full fat ricotta. Season with your salt and pepper.

3. Cut your chicken breasts in half. You want them to still be thick enough to cut pouches into.

4. Carefully cut pockets into one of the ends of each piece of chicken. If you accidentally cut through all the way a little filling might squeeze out, but it's not a big deal. Stuff the pockets with your cheese filling.

5. Tightly wrap two slices of your bacon around each piece of chicken. Try and seal up the open end and any holes where filling might seep out. However, don't wrap it so tight that the chicken folds in on itself or you might have difficulty cooking it through.

6. Pan sear the bacon wrapped chicken in a hot skillet. You don't have to brown all the sides equally, because they will be finished off in the oven.

7. Set your pieces of chicken into an oven safe dish while you finish the others.

8. Bake for approximately 35 to 45 minutes until the bacon is well crisped and the chicken is cooked all the way through. The chicken is done when it reaches 165 degrees.

9. Serve and Enjoy!

<u>Nutrition Facts:</u>

Calories: 385

Net Carbs: 2.3 grams

Conclusion

Thanks for reading my book. I hope this keto fat bombs recipe book has provided you with a nice variety of tasty treats to aid you in your ketogenic diet.

www.ingramcontent.com/pod-product-compliance
Lightning Source LLC
Chambersburg PA
CBHW051045250726
48656CB00001B/149